Fast Track Surgery:
General, Vascular
and Urology

PasTest

Dedicated t

Also by Manoj Ramachandran:

Intercollegiate MRCS: An Aid to the Viva Examination (with Alex Malone and Christopher Chan) published by PasTest.
The Medical Miscellany (with Max Ronson) published by Hammersmith Press.
Clinical Cases and OSCEs in Surgery (with Adam Poole) published by Churchill Livingstone.

Coming soon from Manoj Ramachandran:

Basic Orthopaedic Sciences: The Stanmore Guide published by Hodder Arnold.

Coming soon from Aaron Trinidade and Manoj Ramachandran:

Mnemonics in Surgery published by PasTest.
Fast Track Surgery: Trauma, Orthopaedics, and the Subspecialities published by PasTest.

Fast Track Surgery: General, Vascular and Urology

by

Aaron Trinidade MBBS MRCS(Ed)
Senior House Officer in Otolaryngology, Whipps Cross University
Hospital, London

and

Manoj Ramachandran BSc(Hons) MBBS(Hons)
MRCS(Eng) FRCS(Tr&Orth)
Paediatric and Young Adult Orthopaedic Fellow, Royal National
Orthopaedic Hospital Rotation, Stanmore, Middlesex

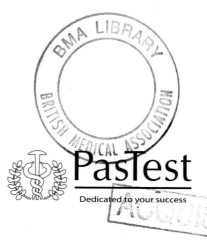

PasTest
Dedicated to your success

© 2006 PASTEST LTD
Egerton Court
Parkgate Estate
Knutsford
Cheshire
WA16 8DX

Telephone: 01565 752000

First published 2006

ISBN: 1904627854

A catalogue record for this book is available from the British Library.

The information contained within this book was obtained by the author from reliable sources. However, while every effort has been made to ensure its accuracy, no responsibility for loss, damage or injury occasioned to any person acting or refraining from action as a result of information contained herein can be accepted by the publishers or author.

PasTest Revision Books and Intensive Courses

PasTest has been established in the field of postgraduate medical education since 1972, providing revision books and intensive study courses for doctors preparing for their professional examinations.

Books and courses are available for the following specialties:

MRCGP, MRCP Parts 1 and 2, MRCPCH Parts 1 and 2, MRCPsych, MRCS, MRCOG Parts 1 and 2, DRCOG, DCH, FRCA, PLAB Parts 1 and 2.

For further details contact:

PasTest, Freepost, Knutsford, Cheshire WA16 7BR
Tel: 01565 752000   Fax: 01565 650264
www.pastest.co.uk   enquiries@pastest.co.uk

Text prepared by Type Study, Scarborough, North Yorkshire
Printed and bound in the UK by Cambridge University Press, Cambridge, UK

CONTENTS

SECTION 1

SECTION 2

ACKNOWLEDGEMENTS

I must firstly thank my parents Austin and Lorna, who have supported me throughout this endeavour, and to whom this book is dedicated. I would like to thank the surgeons who have taught (and grilled) me throughout my profession thus far, and in particular, two of my earlier mentors, Mr Steve Budhooram and Mr Patrick Harnarayan. It is from their often nerve-wracking question and answer sessions that this book sprung, and under their tutelage that I developed the foundation of my surgical knowledge. Stacey, Adrian, and Joelle, thank you for your continuing interest, support, and encouragement. Thanks to PasTest for taking this project on board. Finally, thanks to the many students whom I have had the pleasure of teaching since graduating from medical school. They have brought to me the questions that their own consultants have asked them, and have given me further insight into what they, today's medical students, are expected to know.

Aaron Trinidade

As always, I would first like to thank my wife, Joanna. She has been my inspiration and constant source of support. My parents and my brother, Navin, also deserve special mention. PasTest and in particular, Kirsten Baxter, have been very supportive of all my projects, numerous that they are. I don't think they really know what they've let themselves in for . . .

Manoj Ramachandran

Dear student,

This book was written specifically with you in mind. Your comments, suggestions and corrections are appreciated. If you would like to submit questions you've been asked or mnemonics of your own, we will gladly consider them. If we include it in the next edition of the book, we will add your name on a list of student contributors (good for your curriculum vitae!). In this way, it will truly become your book too! E-mail us at: fasttracksurgery@pastest.co.uk

Aaron Trinidade
Manoj Ramachandran

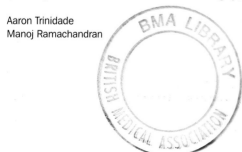

FOREWORD

Current surgical training is very structured, and requires junior surgeons to rapidly acquire knowledge and understanding of surgical practice, prior to progressing into higher surgical training. This is formalised in the MRCS exam. *Fast Track Surgery: General, Vascular, Urology* is an invaluable resource in achieving this aim. The book focuses on solid surgical principles with a structured approach to learning. This allows the junior surgeon to clearly appreciate essential points in patient care.

Broad knowledge, empathy and attention to detail are fundamental to the delivery of good patient care. Early in one's career, the required knowledge base may seem daunting. However a good understanding of basic surgical principles provides a solid foundation to care and facilitates further learning. This book highlights essential knowledge and provides a clear structured method of learning. This mirrors the teaching of basic surgical skills in the apprenticeship style training of good surgical technique. A solid foundation in both of these arms of surgery leads to the development of a competent surgeon. Moreover, it is this foundation that allows competent surgeons to develop into exceptional specialists.

More pressure is now placed upon the training process, to concentrate and condense this training. Attention and stress to structured learning, and the use of general principles and frameworks facilitates this process.

Ultimately the mark of a good surgeon is judgement, both in diagnosis and investigation, and particularly judgement in surgical care. This is the part of our profession that allows us to practise the art of surgery.

The authors of this book are enthusiastic, well motivated surgeons. It has been a pleasure to work with them. They have an excellent surgical understanding, and this is reflected in this clear, concise instructional book in surgical care.

It is a privilege to be a doctor and to be fundamental to care of our patients. With this comes a sincere responsibility to provide excellent surgical care. Personal improvement in provision of patient care is an ongoing task. This we all strive to achieve, through ongoing training, experience, study and research. This book provides a good foundation to understanding principles of care and facilitates the learning of the art of surgery.

Michael Papesch FRACS
Consultant ENT Surgeon
Whipps Cross University Hospital NHS Trust
Leytonstone, London

CONTRIBUTORS

Judith Pearson, MBChB MRCS(Glas)
Registrar in General Practice, St George's Rotation, Bridge Lane Practice, Battersea

Chapter 22: Abdominal aortic aneurysm: leakage and rupture
Chapter 31: Vascular disease

Azhar Ahmad Khan, MBBS MRCS(Ed)
Research Fellow in Urology, Bristol Urology Institute, Southmead Hospital, Bristol

Chapter 34c: Prostate
Chapter 44: Renal carcinoma
Chapter 46: Prostatic carcinoma

Syed Gilani, MBBS MS MRCS(Ed)
Senior House Officer in ITU, Good Hope Hospital, Birmingham

Chapter 28: Abdominal wall: herniae

Mark Prempeh, MBBS MRCS(Glas)
Senior House Officer in Burns & Plastics, Selly Oak Hospital, Birmingham

Chapter 49: Skin cancer

Daniel Horner, BSc MBBS
Senior House Officer in Accident & Emergency, Royal Albert Edward Infirmary, Wigan

Chapter 11: The trauma call

James Stuart Taylor, BSc MBBS
Senior House Officer in Urology, University College of London Hospital, London

Chapter 6: Post-operative complications
Chapter 8: Minimal access surgery

Andrew Skingsley, BSc MBBS
Senior House Officer in ITU/Anaesthetics, Guy's & St Thomas' Hospital,
London

Chapter 7: Anaesthesia

Jodie Lam, BSc MBBS
Senior House Officer ITU/Anaesthetics, Manly Hospital, Sydney, Australia

Chapter 32: Benign breast disease
Chapter 37: Gastric carcinoma
Chapter 43: Breast cancer
Chapter 45: Bladder carcinoma

Charan Koka, BSc MBBS
Senior House Officer in General Practice, Royal Sussex County Hospital,
Brighton

Chapter 35: Skin: lumps and bumps

Amit Parmar, BSc MBBS
House Officer in General Surgery, Whipps Cross University Hospital,
London

Chapter 41: Hepatic carcinoma
Chapter 50: Lymphomas and Sarcomas

SECTION 1

Introduction

USING THIS BOOK AND STUDYING FOR SURGERY

This book was written for you, the medical student on surgical rotations, by registrars and senior house officers (people who are not too far off from where you are right now). Its aim is to serve as a summary of common surgical conditions you are likely to come across during that time. It serves as a rapid-access study aid and is not meant to be a complete surgical text.

Surgery is a logical and practical science, and studying it should be the same. Ideally, after seeing a case on the ward, you should read about it extensively in your standard surgical text and then use this book to refresh and highlight salient points and concepts. Reading should be done daily (or nightly!). The average surgical attachment is approximately 10 weeks. That equates to 70 days. Reading an average of 10 pages a day (approximately 1 hours worth of reading), and 20 a day on Saturday and Sunday mornings from a standard surgical textbook (and this one!), equals 900 pages by the end of the rotation: enough to give you a broad, sound base of surgical knowledge and still leaving adequate time to go on take, and even squeeze in a social life (just about). Sorted!

The book is designed in a question-and-answer type format, and makes use of questions commonly asked on the wards, with the answers given in the succinct and structured way they should be answered. The questions are largely derived from what the authors remember being asked when they were medical students themselves. Applied anatomy is included where relevant (an essential survival tool in the operating theatre!). The book also makes use of tables and mnemonics where appropriate, and gives management plans in list form as you might see written in patients' notes. Blood investigations and radiology are listed *with explanations on why they are ordered*, as the reasons usually evade medical students! Keep this book with you at all times during your clerkship and use it for a bit of cramming from it in your spare moments on the wards. Its two-columned format makes it useful for revision as the answers can be covered up while you test yourself with the questions.

When studying surgery, the following mnemonic is useful to keep in mind:

Dressed **I**n **A** **S**urgeon's **G**own, **A** **P**hysician **I**s **T**ruly **P**rogressing:

Definition
Incidence
Age Distribution
Sex
Geography
Aetiology
Presentation
Investigations
Treatment
Prognosis

This will form a framework on which to build your understanding of each case. The best way to learn is, of course, to clerk patients continuously, no matter how dull it may seem at times. Patients are a wealth of information. Following up the patient reveals investigations performed and management decisions made. This serves to bring to life what you've read and reinforces this information in your mind. But most of all, enjoy your time in surgery – medical school should be fun!

SURVIVING THE SURGICAL ROTATION

The surgical clerkship can be a hectic time. Stress can run high, especially in the operating theatre. The following tips will help you to cope and make the most out of your experience amongst surgeons.

APPEARANCE

Dress smartly and make an effort to appear neat. You will see hundreds of patients, but the patients only see a few of you. White coats help, but be willing to take yours off if it makes a patient anxious (white coat hypertension). Remember you're on a ward dealing with patients, and not in a fashion show. Conservative is always better.

ATTITUDE

You *must* be a keener, but in measured amounts so as not to nauseate fellow students and junior doctors! Strike a balance. A lacklustre attitude leads to lacklustre teaching. Develop thick skin quickly. Sarcasm is common in surgery. Take things in your stride, not personally (unless it was meant to be personal). Be polite, especially to the ward sister who runs the show. Offer to do jobs. Speak up when spoken to, but never backchat. Humility is a virtue. If you can't be humble with your knowledge (or lack thereof), be confident with caution, but *never* cocky. Share information with colleagues and never show others up. Keep skiving to a minimum and make sure everyone pulls his or her weight: the adage 'one bad apple spoils the whole lot' rings true where most busy consultant surgeons are concerned, and you'll then have to really shine to avoid being grouped with slackers.

WHAT TO CARRY

Have the following handy at all times:

- Notebook and pen (have one extra for junior doctors)
- Stethoscope
- Penlight (handy for lumps and bumps)
- Blood and X-ray forms
- This book!

FIRST THING IN THE MORNING, DON'T LOITER!

- Make sure you're there first and say good morning to nursing staff
- Update your personal list of the firm's patients (new admissions, etc)
- Check patients' vitals, blood results and X-rays and have them handy
- Ask the nurses if anything happened overnight
- Have blank blood and X-ray forms handy for the ward round (unless the hospital ordering system is digitalised).

PRESENTING ON THE WARD ROUND

Presenting is an art form to try and perfect. Keep focused and present relevant positives and salient negatives only, but be prepared to answer any question asked (eg knowing who an elderly woman with rectal bleeding lives with is important but need not be presented in the same breath as her current clinical status!). During a presentation, events should be given in a chronological sequence. The following is an example of how a patient should be presented:

[Ms SP, acute appendicitis]

'This is Ms SP, a 26-year-old diabetic secretary who presented at 8 o'clock last night with a 1-day history of worsening abdominal pain radiating from her umbilicus to her right iliac fossa. She described the pain as constant, being aggravated with movement and coughing. Paracetamol did not help. There has been associated nausea, fever and anorexia, but no vomiting. Important negatives include no vaginal discharge or bleeding and no urinary symptoms. Her last normal menstrual period was on [date] and a urinary pregnancy test confirmed that she is not pregnant. Examination revealed a temperature of 38°C and a tachycardia of 95 bpm. All other obs were normal. Abdominal exam revealed a flat abdomen with a Pfannensteil incision from a previous C-section. There was maximal tenderness in the right iliac fossa. There was localised rebound and guarding. Rovsing's sign was positive. Rectal exam revealed nothing of note. A clinical diagnosis of acute appendicitis was made, which was supported by a WBC count of 14. She has been started on antibiotics, analgesia, intravenous fluids, a sliding scale of insulin, and has been NBM since [time]. This morning her vitals are stable [quote values]. She is due for an appendicectomy at [time].'

Presentation time is about 5 minutes, giving plenty of time for questions!

OPERATING THEATRE: DO'S AND DON'TS

DO have a good night's sleep and a proper breakfast before attending
DO review the relevant anatomy beforehand
DO ask the theatre sister to teach you how to scrub up properly (arrive early for this)
DO know the patients inside out *before* they arrive
DO make sure that there is a medical student scrubbed for *every* case
DO use time between cases wisely by either reviewing cases or practising knots
DON'T disturb the surgeon without asking permission first
DON'T annoy the scrub nurse: do as she says
DON'T chit-chat with other students during an operation if not scrubbed
DON'T touch instruments unless given explicit instruction to do so
DON'T look bored no matter how long and tedious the operation is.

POST-OPERATIVE ROUND

If asked to present a patient on post-op rounds, don't panic. Start by stating the procedure the patient had and then use the following list of things that you should be interested in post-operatively:

- General clinical status of patient (alert, vomiting or in pain?)
- Examination (in particular, wound site, chest, calves and bowel sounds)
- Vital signs (look at trends as opposed to single values)
- Fluid charting and input–output balance (is the patient producing urine?)
- Stomas and drains (function and contents)
- Post-operative blood results
- Drug chart (receiving appropriate medications in the appropriate dosages?)

Have gloves for everyone handy in your pockets. Always be the first one to pick up the nursing chart and make a show of checking the vitals. Ask if wounds need to be observed, and if so, take the initiative to remove the dressing yourself (don't forget gloves!). Have your stethoscope handy as surgeons rarely carry one!

Getting started:
THE BASICS

CHAPTER 1: SURGICAL JARGON

a. SURGICAL ABBREVIATIONS

#	Fracture
1ry, 2ry, etc . . .	Primary, Secondary, etc . . .
a/aa	Artery/arteries
AA	Alcoholics Anonymous
AAA	Abdominal aortic aneurysm (triple A)
ABG	Arterial blood gas
Abx	Antibiotics
ABPI	Ankle-brachial pressure index
ADH	Antidiuretic hormone
AF	Atrial fibrillation
AKA	Above knee amputation
Amp	Ampicillin
APR	Abdomino-perineal resection
ARDS	Adult respiratory distress syndrome
ASA	Amino-salicylic acid (aspirin)
ASIS	Anterior superior iliac spine
AXR	Abdominal X-ray
Ba	Barium
bd	*bis die* (twice daily)
BKA	Below knee amputation
BP	Blood pressure
BS	Bowel sounds
CA	Carcinoma
CABG	Coronary artery bypass graft (cabbage)
CBD	Common bile duct
CCF	Congestive cardiac failure
Cef	Cefuroxime
chrm	Chromosome
CIS	Carcinoma in situ
CMV	Cytomegalovirus
C/O	Complains of
COPD	Chronic obstructive pulmonary disease
CPAP	Continuous positive airway pressure
CRP	C-reactive protein (inflammatory marker)

CVA	Cerebrovascular accident (stroke is a better term)
CVP	Central venous pressure
CXR	Chest X-ray
D5W	Dextrose 5% in water
DKA	Diabetic ketoacidosis
DIC	Disseminated intravascular coagulation
DIP	Distal interphalangeal
DRE	Digital rectal examination
DM	Diabetes mellitus
DT	Delirium tremens
DU	Duodenal ulcer
DVT	Deep vein thrombosis
Dx	Diagnosis
ECG	Electrocardiogram
Echo	Echocardiogram
ERCP	Endoscopic retrograde cholangiopancreatography
ESR	Erythrocyte sedimentation rate
ETOH	Alcohol
EUA	Examination under anaesthesia
FAP	Familial adenomatous polyposis
FBC	Full blood count
FDP	Fibrin degradation products
FFP	Fresh frozen plasma
FNA[C]	Fine needle aspirate [cytology]
GA	General anaesthetic
GCS	Glasgow Coma Scale
Gent	Gentamicin
GP	General practitioner
G&S	Group and save
GTN	Glyceryl trinitrate
GU	Genitourinary
GXM	Group and cross-match
HNPCC	Hereditary non-polyposis colorectal cancer
HONK	Hyper-osmolar non-ketotic hyperglycaemic coma

HRT	Hormone replacement therapy
HTN	Hypertension
HIV	Human immunodeficiency virus
HPV	Human papilloma virus
IBD	Inflammatory bowel disease
ICP	Intracranial pressure
I&D	Incision and drainage (abscesses)
IHD	Ischaemic heart disease
ITU	Intensive therapy unit
IMV	Intermittent mandatory ventilation
IPPV	Intermittent positive pressure ventilation
IRV	inverse ratio ventilation/inspiratory reserve volume
IVC	Inferior vena cava
IVDU	Intravenous drug user
IVF	Intravenous fluids
IVP/U	Intravenous pyelogram/urogram
JVP	Jugular venous pressure
KUB	Kidneys, ureters and bladder (plain film)
LA	Local anaesthetic
LAP	Laparotomy
LAP APPY	Laparoscopic appendicectomy
LAP CHOLE	Laparoscopic cholecystectomy
LBO	Large bowel obstruction
LFT	Liver function test
LIF	Left iliac fossa
LIH	Left inguinal hernia
LNMP	Last normal menstrual period
LUQ/LLQ	Left upper/lower quadrant
M/C/S	Microscopy, culture and sensitivity
MEN	Multiple endocrine neoplasia
Metro	Metronidazole
MI	Myocardial infarction
MOF	Multiorgan failure
MSU	Mid-stream urine
n/nn	Nerve/nerves
N/A	Not applicable

NAD	Nil abnormality detected
NBM	Nil by mouth
NGT	Nasogastric tube
NOF	Neck of femur
N/S	Normal saline
NSAIDs	Non-steroidal anti-inflammatory drugs
OCP	Oral contraceptive pill
od	*omni die* (once daily)
OGD	Oesophagogastroduodenoscopy
ORIF	Open reduction and internal fixation
OT	Operating theatre/occupational therapist
PCA	Patient-controlled analgesia
PCWP	Pulmonary capillary wedge pressure
PE	Pulmonary embolism
PEEP	Positive end expiratory pressure
PEG	Percutaneous endoscopic gastrostomy
PERLA	Pupils equal and reactive to light and accommodation
PID	Pelvic inflammatory disease
PIP	Proximal interphalangeal
PO	*per os* (orally)
PR	*per rectum* (rectally)
PRN	*pro re nata* (as needed)
PTC	Percutaneous transhepatic cholangiogram
PTCA	Percutaneous transluminal coronary angioplasty
PUD	Peptic ulcer disease
PUJ	Pelvi-ureteric junction
PV	*per vaginum* (vaginally)
qds	*quater die sumendus* (to be taken 4 times daily)
qxh	every x hours (eg q3h = every 3 hours)
RBS	Random blood sugar
RIF	Right iliac fossa
RIH	Right inguinal hernia

Rx	Treatment
RTA	Road traffic accident
RUQ/RLQ	Right upper/lower quadrant
SBO	Small bowel obstruction
SCC	Squamous cell carcinoma
SIRS	Systemic inflammatory response syndrome
SLE	Systemic lupus erythematosus
SOB	Shortness of breath
stat	Immediately
SVC	Superior vena cava
Sx	Surgery
SXR	Skull X-ray
TB	Tuberculosis
tds	*ter die sumendus* (to be taken 3 times daily)
TIA	Transient ischaemic attack
TOE	Transoesophageal echocardiogram
TPN	Total parenteral nutrition
TURBT	Transurethral resection of bladder tumour
TURP	Transurethral resection of prostate
UC	Ulcerative colitis
U&Es	Urea and electrolytes (and creatinine)
U/O	Urine output
USS	Ultrasound scan
UTI	Urinary tract infection
v/vv	Vein/veins
Vanc	Vancomycin
VE	Vaginal examination
VUJ	Vesico-ureteric junction
WBC/WCC	White blood cells/white cell count
ZES	Zollinger–Ellison syndrome

b. GLOSSARY OF SURGICAL TERMINOLOGY

Aseptic
Complete absence of disease-causing micro-organisms.

Adhesions
Bowel 'stickiness', usually occurring post-op, and predisposing to bowel obstruction. Can be treated with **adhesiolysis**

Adeno-
Pertaining to glands

Afferent
Toward

Anastomosis
Surgically created connection between two tubular structures (eg bowel, blood vessels, etc)

Angio-
Pertaining to blood vessels

Anomalous
Deviating from the norm

Atelectasis
Alveolar collapse

Atresia
Congenital absence of abnormal narrowing of an opening or lumen (adj. **atretic**)

Bezoar
Swallowed mass of foreign material, usually hair or fibre

Bimanual exam
Vaginal examination

Biopsy
Tissue sample obtained and sent for histopathology

Cachexia
Generalised wasting associated with chronic disease or malignancy (adj. **cachectic**)

Calculus
Stone

Calor
One of the classic signs if inflammation; signifies **warmth**

Caseation
Breakdown of diseased tissue into cheese-like material (adj. **caseous**)

Caudal
Relating to lower part of the body

Cephal-
Pertaining to the head

Chole-
Pertaining to the gallbladder

Choledocho-
Pertaining to the bile duct

Cicatrix
Scar

Colic
Pain which occurs in waves; usually occurs in tubular organs

Colonoscopy
Endoscopic examination of the colon

Coprophagia	Ingestion of faeces; one of the causes of **faecatemesis**
Curettage	Scraping of the internal surface of an organ or body cavity with a spoon-line instrument (**curette**)
Cyst	Abnormal sac lined by epithelium and filled with fluid or semi-solid material
Diaphoresis	Excessive sweating
Diverticulum	A small sac or pouch projection from the wall of a hollow organ. The wall of a **true diverticulum** comprises all the layers of the parent organ (eg Meckel's diverticulum). The wall of a **pseudo-diverticulum** contains only some of the layers (eg diverticular disease of the colon)
Dolor	One of the classic signs of inflammation; signifies **pain**
Dysphagia	Difficulty swallowing (as opposed to **odynophagia** which is **painful** swallowing)
Dyspareunia	Painful sexual intercourse (in females)
Ecchymosis	Bruising
-ectomy	Surgical removal (eg cholecystectomy)
Entero-	From **enteric**; pertaining to bowel
Epistaxis	Nosebleed
Excision biopsy	Biopsy in which entire tumour is removed
Faecatemesis	Vomiting of faeces (seen only in **gastrocolic fistula** and **coprophagia**)
Faeculent	Pertaining to faeces (NB faeculent vomiting *resembles* faeces in smell and colour due to intestinal floral action, but is *not* stool as in faecatemesis)
Fistula	An abnormal, **epithelialised** communication between two surfaces

Frequency	Abnormally increased rate of urination
Functio laesa	One of the classic signs of inflammation; signifies **loss of function**
Haemangiona	Benign tumour of blood vessels
Haematemesis	Vomiting of blood
Haematoma	Blood clot within tissues which forms a solid mass. May resolve or become super-infected
Haematuria	Blood in the urine
Haemoptysis	Coughing-up of blood
Haemothorax	Blood within the pleural space
Hesitancy	Difficulty in initiating urination
Icterus	Jaundice
Incisional biopsy	Biopsy in which only a core of the tumour is removed
Induration	Abnormal hardening of a tissue or organ
Intussusception	Telescoping of one part of the bowel into adjacent bowel
Laparotomy	Opening the abdominal cavity via a surgical incision
Laparoscopy	Visualisation of peritoneal cavity with a laparoscope (makes use of fibre optics)
Lumen	Cavity within a tubular organ (adj. **luminal**)
Melaena	Black, tarry stool representing digested blood, most commonly occurring due to an upper GI bleed (must be more than 100 ml)
Nocturia	Abnormal urination at night usually interrupting sleep
Obstipation	Total failure to pass either flatus or stool
Odynophagia	Painful swallowing
Orchid-	Pertaining to the testicles
-orraphy	Surgical repair (eg herniorraphy)

-oscopy	Visual examination of the interior of the abdomen (through an endoscope)
-ostomy	Surgically created opening (eg colostomy). (From *stoma* which means mouth)
-otomy	Surgical incision into an organ (eg laparostomy)
-pexy	Surgical fixation (eg orchidopexy)
Phlegmon	Solid, swollen, inflamed pancreatic tissue mass
Pneumaturia	Air in the urine (usually due to an **enterovesical fistula**)
Pneumothorax	Air within the pleural space
Pus	Fluid product of inflammation (see Chapter 24) (Adj. **purulent**, *not* pussy!)
Rubor	One of the classic signs of inflammation; signifies **redness**
Sinus	Abnormal, blind-ending, epithelialised tract in an organ
Steatorrhoea	Fatty stools due to decreased fat absorption
Stenosis	Abnormal narrowing of a lumen, passage or opening
Strangury	A painful discharge of urine, drop by drop, caused by spasmodic bladder contraction
Succus entericus	Fluid from the bowel lumen
Suppuration	Formation of pus
Tenesmus	Sensation of rectal fullness with urge to defecate
Transection	Transverse division
Urgency	Sudden urge to urinate

c. SURGICAL SIGNS, TESTS, LAWS, SYNDROMES AND EPONYMS

Aaron's sign	Pressure in RIF causes epigastric and cardiac discomfort in chronic appendicitis
Afferent loop syndrome	Chronic obstruction of duodenum and jejunum proximal to gastrojejunostomy performed in Billroth II procedure
Allen's test	Test of hand circulation. Ask pt. to drain hand by forming a fist, and compress radial and ulnar aa. Ask pt. to open blanched fist. Release one artery and observe for palmar flushing (arterial patency). Repeat test for other artery
Battle's sign	Periorbital ecchymoses in basal skull #
Beck's triad	Seen in cardiac tamponade. Consists of: 1. Jugular venous distension 2. Muffled heart sounds 3. ↓BP
Boas' sign	Right subscapular pain in cholelithiasis
Boerhaave's syndrome	Oesophageal rupture (traumatic or after binge drinking)
Carcinoid syndrome	Syndrome caused by serotonin release from carcinoid tumour. Consists of: 1. Bronchospasm 2. Flushing 3. Diarrhoea 4. Right-sided heart failure
Charcot's triad	Seen in ascending cholangitis. Consists of:

1. Fever with rigors
2. Jaundice
3. RUQ pain

Chvostek's sign

Seen in hypocalcaemia. Tapping over facial n. causes twitching of facial muscles

Compartment syndrome

Condition of increased pressure in a confined anatomical space adversely affecting circulation and threatening the function and viability of tissues therein

Courvoisier's law

'If, in the presence of jaundice, a mass is present in the right upper quadrant, the jaundice is unlikely to be due to stones.' (The cause is therefore most likely carcinoma of pancreatic head, since in gallstones the gallbladder is **fibrotic and shrivelled**)

Cullen's sign

Periumbilical ecchymosis 2ry to retroperitoneal haemorrhage (as seen in haemorrhagic pancreatitis)

Cushing's triad

Seen in raised ICP. Consists of:
1. ↑BP
2. Bradycardia
3. Irregular respirations

Cushing's syndrome

Clinical syndrome of glucocorticoid excess. If due to excess ACTH levels (as in pituitary tumour or ectopic production), known as **Cushing's disease**

Dercum's disease

Multiple, painful lipomatosis (mainly truncal)

Dumping syndrome

Seen after gastric vagotomy, pyloroplasty and gastrojejunostomy. Caused by rapid passage of large amounts of hyperosmolar chyme into small bowel. Consists of:

1. Autonomic instability (flushing, sweating, dizziness, vasomotor collapse)
2. Abdominal pain
3. Diarrhoea

Fox's sign

Inguinal ligament ecchymosis 2ry to retroperitoneal haemorrhage (as seen in haemorrhagic pancreatitis)

Gardner's syndrome

Autosomal dominant premalignant syndrome consisting of:

1. Multiple colonic polyposis
2. Skull osteomas
3. Epidermoid cysts
4. Fibromas

Goodsall's line and law

Line: imaginary line drawn horizontally through the anus of a patient in the lithotomy position.
Law: anal fistulae occurring above this line (anterior fistulae) take a straight course to the anal canal; those below it (posterior fistulae) take a curved course

Grey Turner's sign

Flank ecchymosis seen in retroperitoneal haemorrhage (as seen in haemorrhagic pancreatitis).
Mnemonic: Turner = turn pt. on side = flank

Homan's sign

Seen in DVT. Calf pain on foot dorsiflexion. Dangerous (may dislodge a clot!) and rarely used

Kaposi–Stemmer sign

Inability to pick up or pinch a fold of skin in lymphoedema

Kehr's sign

Intense left shoulder tip pain in splenic rupture. Caused by referred pain due to diaphragmatic irritation

Krukenburg tumour	Metastatic tumour to ovary, classically from stomach
Leriche's syndrome	Seen in iliac occlusive disease. Consists of: 1. Buttock claudication 2. Buttock atrophy 3. Impotence
McBurney's point and sign	**Point:** Starting from the umbilicus, a point 2/3 along a line drawn from the umbilicus to the right ASIS **Sign:** Pressure on this point causes pain in acute appendicitis
Mendelson's syndrome	Chemical aspiration pneumonitis following aspiration of gastric contents
Mirrizi's syndrome	Extraluminal compression of CBD from a cystic gallstone. May cause obstructive jaundice
Murphy's sign	Seen in cholecystitis. Palpation of RUQ causes pain on inspiration as inflamed gallbladder moves downward and 'hits' the palpating hand
Obturator sign	Seen in appendicitis and pelvic abscess. Pain on internal rotation of right lower limb with knee and hip flexed
Ogilvie's syndrome	Massive **non-obstructive** colonic dilation. Syn: **pseudo-obstruction**
Panda eyes	See **Raccoon eyes**
Peutz–Jegher's syndrome	Syndrome of benign GI polyps with circumoral pigmentation
Plummer–Vinson syndrome	Syndrome of the oesophageal webs and dysphagia caused by iron deficiency. May develop into SCC (10%)

Psoas sign	Seen in appendicitis and psoas inflammation. Pain on extending the hip with knee in full extension
Raccoon eyes	Seen in basal skull #. Bilateral periorbital ecchymoses. Syn: **Panda eyes**
Refeeding syndrome	$\downarrow$K, $\downarrow$Mg and $\downarrow$PO$_4$ following refeeding of a starved patient
Reynold's pentad	Seen in suppurative cholangitis. Consists of: 1. Fever with rigors 2. Jaundice 3. RUQ pain 4. CNS alteration 5. Shock/sepsis (Basically Charcot's triad + 2)
Rovsing's sign	Seen in appendicitis. Palpation in LIF causes pain in RIF.
Saint's triad	3 conditions which usually co-exist. If you find 1, look for other 2: 1. Cholelithiasis 2. Hiatal hernia 3. Diverticular disease
Short-gut syndrome	Malnutrition resulting from <100 cm of viable small bowel
Sipple syndrome	MEN II
Sister Mary Joseph's sign	Metastatic tumour to umbilical lymph node(s)
Superior vena cava syndrome	SVC obstruction (eg by tumour, thrombosis) causing engorged face, neck and upper chest veins (SVC distribution)
Thoracic outlet syndrome	Compression of structures exiting thoracic outlet (eg cervical rib)
Tietze's syndrome	Costochondritis of rib cartilages presenting as pleuritic-type pain. Aseptic. Treat with NSAIDs

Trousseau's sign	Seen in hypocalcaemia. Carpopedal spasm after blood occlusion (with BP cuff) in forearm or leg
Trousseau's syndrome	Syndrome of DVT associated with carcinoma
Virchow's node	Metastatic tumour to left supraclavicular node(s)
von Hippel–Lindau syndrome	An autosomal dominant syndrome of retinal and cerebellar angiomata occasionally associated with renal cell carcinoma and phaeochromocytoma
Werner's syndrome	MEN I
Whipple's triad	Seen in insulinoma. Consists of: 1. Hypoglycaemia 2. CNS and vasomotor symptoms (syncope and diaphoresis) 3. Symptomatic relief following glucose administration
Zollinger–Ellison's syndrome	Syndrome of gastrinoma and PUD

CHAPTER 2: INCISIONS

Figure 2.1 Incisions

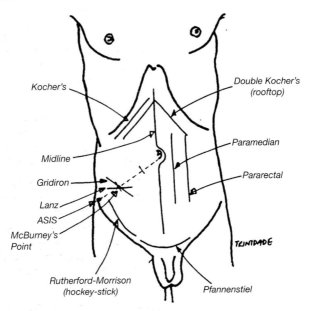

Kocher's

Double Kocher's (rooftop)

Paramedian

Midline

Pararectal

Gridiron

Lanz

ASIS

McBurney's Point

TRINIDADE

Rutherford-Morrison (hockey-stick)

Pfannenstiel

What comprises an ideal abdominal incision?

It should:
- Allow easy and rapid access
- Be easily extendible
- Heal securely (hence avoiding **dehiscence** and **herniae**)
- Be relatively pain free post-op
- Appear cosmetically pleasing.

What incisions do you know of?

Midline: made through **linea alba**, hence relatively bloodless; used for most laparotomies (also **upper** and **lower** midline incisions).

Paramedian: made through **rectus abdominis** ≈1.5 cm from midline; intercostal nerves may be divided. Higher risk of bleeding and herniae. Used in upper GI surgery.

Pararectal: made just lateral to rectus. No longer used due to high risk of intercostal damage.

Kocher's: made 3 cm below right costal margin from midline to edge of rectus sheath; used in biliary surgery (eg cholecystectomy). Can be used on the left side of the abdomen for splenectomy.

Double Kocher's (rooftop): basically a left and right-sided Kocher's joining in the midline; used in pancreatic and gastric surgery.

Gridiron: made through **McBurney's point** (see p. 26) at right angles to McBurney's line; used in appendicectomy. Risk of dividing **iliohypogastric nerve** medially, resulting in **direct inguinal hernia** (due to weakening of **conjoint tendon**).

Lanz: modification of gridiron, but transversely. More cosmetic result as made along **Langer's lines** (natural skin creases).

Pfannenstiel: transverse lower abdominal incision; used extensively in gynaecological and pelvic surgery. Lowest incidence of incisional herniae.

Rutherford–Morrison (hockey-stick): external oblique splitting incision affording good access to caecum, appendix and right colon. Mainly used during kidney transplant surgery (donor kidney usually transplanted into RIF).

CHAPTER 3: WOUNDS, STOMAS, FISTULAE, ANASTOMOSES, TUBES AND DRAINS

WOUNDS

How can wounds be classified?

Incised: relatively clean, caused by sharp object (Rx: 1ry suture).
Lacerated: contaminated with jagged edges, as seen post RTA (Rx: edge excision and 1ry suture).
Crushed and devitalised: seen mostly in severe RTA and industrial accidents (Rx: debridement and healing by 2ry intention if contaminated or dirty).

How else can wounds be classified?

Clean, as in hernia surgery (no viscus breached)
Clean contaminated, as in elective GI surgery (viscus breached, insignificant spillage).
Contaminated, as in bowel perforation (gross spillage, but no pus/gangrene).
Dirty, as in pelvic abscess (frank pus/gangrene encountered).

How do wounds heal?

By **primary** or **secondary** intention
Healing by **primary intention** occurs if wound edges are brought together immediately. Scarring is minimal.
Healing by **secondary intention** occurs if wound edges are not brought together (irreparable skin loss, wound infection, wound breakdown). Wound defect fills up with **granulation tissue** from the base upwards. Slower than primary intention and produces more scarring.

What factors have an adverse effect on wound healing?

mnemonic: **VITAMINS A, B, C, D, E**
Vitamin deficiency
Infection (local and generalised)
Technique
Arterial supply (especially vascular disease or trauma)
Malnutrition
Icterus (2ry to hepatobiliary disease, haemolysis or uraemia)
Necrotic tissue
Sugar (diabetes mellitus)
Anaemia, **A**ge
Blood clot (haematoma formation)
Cancer (local or distant)
Drugs (cytotoxic agents and steroids)
Edge tension (esp. in **obesity**).

What abnormalities in scarring do you know of?

Hypertrophic scarring: excessive scarring which *remains within* the margins of the wound edges. Common in the young and after burns. (Rx: compression).
Keloid formation: excessive scarring which *extends beyond* the wound edges. Common in dark-skinned races and in certain anatomical regions (sternum, deltoid). (Rx: difficult as high recurrence rate; steroid impregnation. Excision makes condition worse on recurrence). (Syn. **proud flesh.**)

STOMAS

What is a stoma?

An artificial opening of the gut which has been brought to the abdominal surface.

What type of stomas do you know of?

1. Gastrostomy
2. Jejunostomy
3. Ileostomy
4. Caecostomy
5. Colostomy.

What are the indications for stoma formation?

mnemonic: **FLEDD**

Feeding: gastrostomy, jejunostomy (eg post GI surgery or in CNS disease)

Lavage: caecostomy (eg on-table bowel prep before distal colonic surgery; used rarely)

Exteriorisation: colostomy, ileostomy (see below)

Decompression: caecostomy (in gross bowel obstruction; rarely used now)

Diversion: ileostomy, colostomy (see below), duodenostomy (following duodenal trauma; rare).

What are the differences between an ileostomy and a colostomy?

(See Table 3.1)

Table 3.1

	Ileostomy	**Colostomy**
Site	Usually RIF	Usually LIF
Shape	Spouted. This is due to caustic nature of effluent which irritates surrounding skin (**high enzyme content**). Spout minimises this.	Flat/flush with skin
Effluent	Liquid to semi-liquid (small bowel contents)	Semi-solid to solid (faecal)
Output	**Low output:** 500 ml/day **High output:** 1 litre/day	200–300 ml/day (less with lower colostomies)

When would you use an ileostomy?

Either to protect a distal (colonic) anastomosis (**temporary**) or following **panproctocolectomy** (**permanent**). Also used to rest distal bowel, eg after **right colonic trauma**, **persistent fistulae** or **Crohn's**.

When would a panprocto-colectomy be performed?	1. Ulcerative colitis (UC) 2. Familial adenomatous polyposis coli (FAP) 3. **Severe** Crohn's disease (otherwise, surgical intervention is **conservative**) 4. Multiple colonic cancer.
What types of ileostomies do you know of?	**Loop ileostomy** (temporary) and **terminal/end ileostomy** (usually permanent).
When would you use a colostomy?	Either to protect a distal anastomosis (**temporary**) or following **abdomino-perineal resection** (**permanent**). Also used as a temporary measure after colonic resection if primary anastomosis is not immediately feasible (**temporary**).

Figure 3.1 Terminal ileostomy and types of colostomy

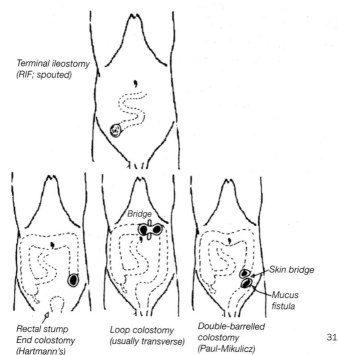

Terminal ileostomy
(RIF; spouted)

Bridge

Skin bridge

Mucus fistula

Rectal stump
End colostomy
(Hartmann's)

Loop colostomy
(usually transverse)

Double-barrelled
colostomy
(Paul-Mikulicz)

31

What types of colostomies do you know of?

Loop colostomy: loop of colon brought to surface and secured with plastic/glass rod; bowel opened and edges sewn to skin. Diversion only. Easily reversible.

End colostomy and rectal stump (Hartmann's procedure): proximal end of colon brought up as end colostomy and distal end is stapled and dropped back into peritoneal cavity. Mucus produced by it passed *per anum*. Reversible but can be difficult (stump may be hard to find).

Double-barrelled colostomy (Paul–Mikulicz procedure): both ends are brought to surface. Proximal end is functional, while distal end is a **mucus fistula** (discharges mucus). Easily reversible.

When would you reverse a a colostomy?

After 6 weeks. After 12 weeks, reversal becomes more difficult due to adhesions.

What are the complications of stomas?

mnemonic: **STOMA BAGS HELP**
Stenosis
Tight defect (*narrow abdominal wall defect leading to* ***ischaemia/gangrene***)
Overflow (of afferent bowel contents into efferent limb; may compromise distal anastomosis)
Maintenance problems (stoma nurse/education helps)
Anaemia (esp. megaloblastic due to terminal ileal loss in ileostomy)
Bloating (flatus may be a problem)
Aroma (malodour helped with deodorants)
Gall/kidney stones (due to loss of terminal ileum/bile salt absorption; and dehydration respectively)
Short-gut syndrome (excess fluid/electrolyte loss)

Hernia *(parastomal)*
Excoriation *(of skin, esp. in ileostomy)*
Leakage *(usually 2ry to ill-fitting device)*
Prolapse *(may need re-fashioning).*

[Not listed in order of importance. Complications in *italics* are **primary**.]

What is an ileal conduit?

A loop of ileum used for urinary diversion, mainly after **cystectomy** (excision of bladder). Both ureters are anastomosed to one end of the loop and the other end is brought to the surface as a spout (**urostomy**). Look for urine in the stoma bag.

FISTULAE

What is a fistula?

An abnormal connection between two epithelial or endothelial structures (the connection occurs within or between organs, vessels, and intestines).

What causes a fistula?

Fistulae are usually the result of injury, surgery, infection or inflammation.

Which disease is renowned for fistula formation?

Crohn's disease.

What type of fistulae do you know of?

1. **Blind:** connects 2 structures, but open on 1 end only
2. **Complete:** has both external and internal openings
3. **Incomplete:** a fistula from the skin that is closed on the inside and does not connect to any internal structure
4. **Horse-shoe:** connects the anus to the surface of the skin after going around the rectum (see Chapter 30).

Can you give some examples?

Examples include:
1. Arteriovenous (artery to vein)
2. Fistula-in-ano (anal canal to skin)
3. Urachal (bladder to skin)
4. Rectovaginal (bowel to vagina)
5. Enterocystic (bowel to bladder)
6. Branchial (branchial cyst to skin)
7. Enterocutaneous (bowel to skin).

What conditions prevent closure of a fistula?

mnemonic: **FRIEND**
Foreign body
Radiation
Infection
Epithelialisation
Neoplasia
Distal obstruction.

How should a fistula be managed?

Depends on the type of fistula, but generally by avoidance of the above. Excision of the fistula may be attempted.

ANASTOMOSES

What is an anastomosis?

A surgically created connection between two normally separate tubular organs or parts.

Where are anastomoses used?

Bowel surgery, vascular surgery, urological surgery and transplant surgery.

In bowel surgery, what is the difference between primary and secondary anastomosis?

Primary anastomosis is performed on the proximal and distal ends of bowel following bowel resection at the initial operation.
Secondary anastomosis is performed at a second operation. A colostomy is usually fashioned in the interim at the initial operation following bowel resection.

When would primary anastomosis not be feasible in bowel surgery?

In the presence of perforation, sepsis, ischaemia, intestinal obstruction or disease at anastomotic site (eg Crohn's). The presence of these increase the risk of anastomotic leakage.

How does a bowel anastomotic leak present?

Usually on day 5 post-op with **pyrexia** and **tachycardia**. Signs of shock may ensue.

TUBES

What type of tubes do you know of?

1. Urinary tract tubes:
   Urinary catheter (urethral and suprapubic). (Syn. **Foley catheter**)
2. Respiratory tract tubes:
   Airway tubes (see p. 36)
   Chest tube
3. Vascular system tubes:
   IV lines (see p. 37)
   Central lines
4. Gastrointestinal system tubes:
   Nasogastric tube
   Flatus tube
   Gastrostomy tube (see above)
   Duodenostomy tube (see above)
   Jejunostomy tube (see above)
5. Biliary tree tubes:
   T-tube cholecystostomy tube.

What does 'French' mean when describing tube size?

It describes diameter. The higher the French (F), the wider the diameter. Divide the French number by π (3.14, or approx. 3) to get diameter in mm (eg 12 F $\approx$ 4 mm)

How does this differ from 'gauge'?

Gauge is used in needle size and represents the fraction of an inch the bore diameter is (eg 16-gauge = 1/16 inch bore) The higher the gauge, the finer the bore (opposite of French).

URINARY TRACT TUBES

What structures does a urethral catheter traverse during male catheterisation?

1. Urethral meatus
2. Penile (spongy) urethra
3. Membranous urethra
4. Prostatic urethra
5. Bladder neck
6. Bladder.

How many lumina does a urinary catheter have?

Either 2 or 3.
A **2-way** catheter has one for urinary diversion and one for balloon inflation. A **3-way** has a 3rd for **bladder irrigation**.

What's the landmark for suprapubic catheter insertion?

1 finger's-breadth above symphysis pubis. Ensure bladder is full (dull percussion; aspirate for urine if unsure).

RESPIRATORY TRACT TUBES

What are the indications for chest tube insertion?

1. Pneumothorax (simple or tension): **air**
2. Haemothorax: **blood**
3. Pneumo-haemothorax: **air and blood**
4. Chylothorax **chyle**
5. Empyema: **pus**
6. Large pleural effusion: **transudate/exudate**.

Where would you insert it?

5th intercostal space in the mid-axillary line.

Would you go over or under a rib with the tube?

Over, to avoid neurovascular bundle on underside of rib.

How do you know you're in the pleural cavity?

By a whoosh of air and moisture forming on the tube.

How should the tube be directed?

Upwards and posteriorly towards the lung apex.

What would you connect it to?	An underwater seal.
What would you look for?	Oscillation (up and down movement of water level with every respiratory cycle) to ensure proper functioning.
What *must* be done post-insertion?	Check CXR to assess positioning and extent of insertion (last hole is cut through radio-opaque line and shows as a break in the line).

VASCULAR SYSTEM TUBES

What is a central line?	A line placed into the right atrium via the internal jugular, subclavian or femoral vein.
What are the indications for central line insertion?	***mnemonic:* CHIPS** **C**VP monitoring, **C**ardiac pacing **H**aemodialysis **I**nfusions (TPN, chemotherapy) **P**ulmonary artery catheterisation **S**hoddy peripheral venous access.
What are the complications?	1. Catheter tip embolus or thrombotic embolus 2. Arrhythmias 3. Pneumothorax 4. Haemothorax 5. Pleural effusion 6. Air embolism 7. Infection 8. Bleeding 9. Subclavian vein thrombosis.
What *must* be done post-insertion?	Check CXR for positioning or evidence of pneumothorax.

GASTROINTESTINAL SYSTEM TUBES

What are the indications for nasogastric tube (NGT) insertion?

1. Emptying of stomach contents (esp. emergency pre-op to avoid aspiration)
2. Rest bowel (eg in pancreatitis)
3. Feeding (use fine bore NGT).

What's the big risk in inserting a nasogastric tube?

Intubating the trachea.

How is this avoided?

By asking the patient to swallow water when tube is at back of throat (epiglottis covers glottis during swallowing.

How can you test the tube is in the stomach?

Insufflate air down tube with a syringe whilst auscultating the stomach (a whoosh of air will be heard), or by aspirating stomach contents back.

What *must* be done before feeding through an NGT?

CXR to r/o intrathoracic placement and hence risk of chemical pneumonitis.

What is a flatus tube?

A large bore, flexible tube used to decompress obstructed large bowel by allowing passage of flatus. It is passed *per rectum*. Used esp. in sigmoid volvulus.

BILIARY TREE TUBES

What is a cholecystostomy tube?

A tube used to drain the gallbladder. Inserted under USS guidance. Placed either surgically or percutaneously.

What is a T-tube?

A tube placed into the biliary tree, usually after it has been surgically explored. It drains bile percutaneously.

What is the minimum amount of time a T-tube must be left in?

10 days. By this time a fibrous tract has formed around the tube which then scleroses on the tube's removal. This prevents bile leakage post-removal.

What factors determine a T-tube is safe to be removed?

Clinically: no signs/symptoms of cholangitis on clamping (see Chapter 16)
Biochemically: no derangement in LFTs on clamping
Radiologically: T-tube cholangiogram is normal.

DRAINS

What are the indications for drainage?

1. Removal of infected foreign material
2. Obliteration of dead space
3. Monitoring (eg for leakage post bowel anastomosis).

What drains do you know of?

Penrose drain: thin, soft rubber tube. Non-traumatic. Used in abscess cavities.
Sheet drain: corrugated drain which drains fluid via a gutter action (eg **Yeates drain**, sheet drain comprising many draining tubes in parallel)
Tube drain: firm Silastic tube with several holes at end. In abdominal surgery, it is connected to a bag forming a **closed system**. In cardiothoracic surgery, an underwater seal is used. Suction machine may be needed.
Vacuum drain: similar to tube drains, but vacuum apparatus applied to end to create negative pressure (eg Redivac, Sterivac). Negates need for suction machine.

CHAPTER 4: FLUID, ELECTROLYTE AND ACID–BASE BALANCE

FLUID BALANCE

What percentage of lean body mass (LBM) is water?

Approximately 60%, which equates to about 42 litres (L), the **total body water (TBW)**, in the average 70 kg man.

What compartments is this water found in?

Intracellular fluid and **extracellular fluid** compartments (ICF and ECF respectively).

How is it divided up?

TBW: 42 L →
ICF: 28 L (66%)
→ ECF: 14 L (33%), subdivided into:
    → Interstitium 11 L (75%)
    → Intravascular 3 L (25%)

How is water balance controlled?

Input controlled via **thirst**. Output controlled via **renin–aldosterone–angiotensin axis** and **ADH**.

Which water compartment fluctuates daily?

The ECF compartment (approx. 2500 ml/day of the total 14 litres) (See Table 4.1).

Table 4.1

ECF (14 litres)	
Input (2500 ml)	**Output (2500 ml)**
	Sensible losses:
Fluid: 1300 ml	Urine: 1500 ml
Food: 800 ml	Faeces: 100 ml
Metabolic water: 400 ml	
	Insensible losses:
	Skin: 500 ml
	Lung: 400 ml

Which means what?	This means that the average 70 kg man requires ≈2500 ml/day (**30–35 ml/kg/day**) of **maintenance fluids** to replace daily losses.
What are the normal salt requirements/day?	Na ≈ 1 mEq/kg/day K ≈ 1 mEq/kg/day Cl ≈ 1.5 mEq/kg/day

In surgical patients, what types of fluid losses do you know of?	1. Sensible and insensible losses (see Table 4.1)
	2. Abnormal losses:
	  a. Gut: diarrhoea, vomiting
	  b. Fever
	  c. Hyperventilation
	  d. Tubes and drains
	  e. 3rd space losses.

What is 3rd space fluid loss?	Fluid lost to **sequestration**. Can occur in areas of trauma and inflammation, and in bowel obstruction (see Chapter 18).
So what must be achieved when prescribing fluids?	1. Correction of pre-existing deficit 2. Fulfilment of daily requirements (maintenance fluids for sensible and insensible losses) 3. Replacement of ongoing abnormal losses (measure if possible).
How can pre-existing deficit be determined?	**History:** Vomiting, diarrhoea, thirst **Examination:** ↓skin turgor, sunken eyes, dry mucous membranes, tachycardia, oliguria **Investigations:** ↑Hct, ↑urea, conc. urine (Osm > 650).
How can the amount of maintenance fluids needed in 24 hours be estimated?	By using the following formula: 100 ml/kg for 1st 10 kg 50 ml/kg for next 10 kg 20 ml/kg for every kg over 20 kg eg in the average 70 kg man, the amount of maintenance fluids needed would be:

$$100 \times 10 = 1000 +$$
$$50 \times 10 = 500 +$$
$$20 \times (70 - 20) = 20 \times 50 = 1000$$
Total: $1000 + 500 + 1000 = 2500$ ml/day (Divide by 24 to get hourly rate).

How is all of this achieved on the ward?

The average person is usually assumed to need a maintenance of ≈3000 ml (3 litres) of fluid/day. This is usually given as 3 bags, each containing 1 litre of fluid. Each bag is run over 8 hours. The amount of fluid can be ↑ or ↓ depending on the clinical situation or the size of the individual (eg children who are *always* given fluids on a ml/kg/hour basis).

What fluids used in clinical practice do you know of?

(See Table 4.2).

Table 4.2*

	Alternative name	Na	Cl	K	HCO$_3$
Sodium chloride 0.9%	Normal saline (N/S)	150	150		
Ringer's lactate	Hartmann's	131	111	5	29 (lactate)
Glucose 5%	5% Dextrose (D5W)				
Glucose 4%, sodium chloride 0.18%	Dextrose saline (D/S)	30	30		

*Commonest fluids used are shown only; all figures represent mmol/L.

What common fluid regimes do you know of?

1. 3 L N/S @ 1 L 8 hourly
2. 2 L N/S + 1 L 5% D/W @ 1 L 8 hourly
3. 3 L D/S @ 1 L 8 hourly

Others exist; common ones shown here.

Which fluid is most commonly used maintenance fluid?	Normal saline with 20 mEq KCl/L
What is the most commonly used resuscitative fluid?	Hartmann's solution.
How is fluid balance monitored?	Via **urine output** (with or without a catheter). In patients with cardiac or renal dysfunction, a CVP line may be more appropriate).
What is the minimal acceptable urinary output?	30 ml/h (maintenance); 50 ml/h (trauma).
Is less maintenance fluid needed post-operatively?	Yes. The trauma of surgery causes release of vasoconstricting substances such as ADH, aldosterone cortisol. These ↓ intravascular volume and hence the need for as much fluid. This is known as the **stress response**.

POTASSIUM BALANCE

HYPERKALAEMIA

What are the causes of ↑K?	*mnemonic:* **HI POTASSIuM**
	Hypoaldosteronism (Addison's disease)
	Iatrogenic (excess K infusion)
	Potassium-sparing diuretics (eg spironolactone)
	Oliguria
	Tissue destruction (rhabdomyolysis, **burns**)
	Acidosis
	Spurious (lab error; very common!)
	Suxamethonium (inducing agent in anaesthesia)
	Ingestion (potassium iodide, bananas, citrus)
	Massive blood transfusion.

How does it present?	Cardiac arrhythmias, sudden death. Look for **tall, tented T-waves** on ECG.
When is it treated?	When K level > 6.5 mmol/L and there are ECG changes (make sure and r/o spurious value!)
What is the treatment?	*Treat underlying cause, then:* Remember: **10–10–20–50–50** **10 ml** of a **10%** solution of calcium resonium (**cardioprotective**); give *slowly* over 2 min Follow with: **20 U** of soluble insulin (eg Actrapid); this pushes K into cells. Give with: **50 ml** of a **50%** solution of glucose Follow with a calcium resonium enema to remove GI potassium (**chelating agent**).

HYPOKALAEMIA

What are the causes of ↓K?	*mnemonic:* **CRAMPING** **C**ushing's and **C**onn's syndromes **R**enal tubular failure **A**lkalosis **M**ucus per rectum (**villous adenoma**; important surgical cause!) **P**yloric stenosis **I**ntestinal fistulae **N**G aspiration **G**I upset (vomiting and diarrhoea).
How does it present?	**Cramping**(!), muscle weakness, hypotonia, cardiac arrhythmias. Look for **small** or **inverted** **T-waves** and **U-waves** on ECG.
What is the critical level?	When K < 2.5 mmol/L.
What is the treatment?	*Treat underlying cause, then:* If >2.5 mmol/L, oral supplementation (Sando-K) If <2.5 mmol/L, *slow* IV infusion.

| When would you give a bolus dose of potassium? | **NEVER!** Can cause fatal arrhythmias! (This is a famous trick question!) |

SODIUM BALANCE

HYPERNATRAEMIA

What are the causes of ↑Na?	*mnemonic:* **SALTED** **S**weating **A**ddison's disease **L**ack of fluids (common cause on the wards!) **T**PN **E**mesis (vomiting) **D**iabetes insipidus, **D**ehydration.
How does it present?	Thirst, confusion, coma then seizures. Look for sunken eyes, dry mucous membranes, skin tenting, skin mottling and (in babies) depressed fontanelles.
What is the treatment?	Oral water if possible. Also *slow* D5W or N/S.

HYPONATRAEMIA

| What types of hyponatraemia do you know of? | Hypovolaemic, euvolaemic and hypervolaemic. |
| What are the differences? | (See Table 4.3) |

Table 4.3

	Hypovolaemic	Euvolaemic	Hypervolaemic
Pathophysiology	Both Na and water are lost resulting in a concurrent low blood volume; **normal osmolarity**	Only Na is lost; blood volume remains constant; **hypo-osmolarity**	Blood volume is ↑; Na remains constant; overall effect is **dilutional**; **hypo-osmolarity**
Causes	**Burns** Pancreatitis Diuretic excess NG suction	**SIADH** CNS abnormalities	**Renal failure** CCF Liver failure IV fluid excess
Treatment (after underlying cause is addressed)	IV N/S	In SIADH, N/S and frusemide stat, followed by fluid restriction	Fluid restriction and diuretics

ACID–BASE BALANCE

What is normal pH?

7.40 +/− 0.05 (ie 7.35–7.45)

What regulates pH?

HCO_3, various other buffers (including Hb and other proteins) and the kidney (H^+ regulation) according to the **Henderson–Hasselbach equation:**

$$H^+ + HCO_3^- \leftrightarrow H_2CO_3 \leftrightarrow H_2O + CO_2$$

HCO_3^- is an alkali and CO_2 is an acidic gas.

What type of acid–base disorders do you know?

Metabolic acidosis and alkalosis. Respiratory acidosis and alkalosis.

What is acidosis?

pH < 7.35

What is alkalosis?

pH > 7.45

What makes a disorder metabolic or respiratory?

1ry changes in HCO_3^- are metabolic. 1ry changes in CO_2 are respiratory.

What are normal HCO_3^- and CO_2 values?	HCO_3^-: 22–28 mmol/L CO_2: 4.7–6.0 kPa
How is an ABG interpreted then?	HCO_3^- and CO_2 are the 2 main values to assess. If HCO_3^- is abnormal and in keeping with pH change, the problem is mainly **metabolic.** If CO_2 is abnormal and in keeping with pH change, the problem is mainly **respiratory**. Whether acidotic or alkalotic will now depend on pH. *eg pH = 7.20, HCO_3^- = 12, CO_2 = 4.8* pH is ↓, therefore an acidosis is present. HCO_3^- is ↓ and CO_2 is normal. Therefore it is a metabolic problem. HCO_3^- is an alkali, so a fall will result in acidosis. This is in keeping with pH. This represents a **metabolic acidosis**.

METABOLIC ACIDOSIS

What are the changes?	**↓pH, ↓HCO_3^-**
What are the causes?	Conditions which *either* **cause HCO_3^- loss** from the body, *or* ↑**acids** (and hence H) in the blood, thus causing HCO_3 consumption via the following equation: $$↑H^+ + HCO_3^- \rightarrow H_2CO_3 \rightarrow H_2O + CO_2$$ (gain in H^+ causes a right shift in the equation). Conditions causing an ↑ in H^+ usually cause an ↑ in the **anionic gap**.
What is the anionic gap?	A measure of the presence of anions not usually measured in the lab (ie all excluding Cl and HCO_3^-). Remember that anions bind H^+ to make acids

(eg SO_4^- reversibly binds H^+ to make H_2SO_4, sulphuric acid). An $\uparrow$ anion gap means $\uparrow$ levels of anions in the blood which are donating their H^+ ions and causing acidosis (eg ketones in ketoacidosis and lactate in lactic acidosis).

The anion gap is measured with the following:

$$[Na^+ + K^+] - [HCO_3^- + Cl^-]$$

What is the normal anion gap?

11–19 mmol/L

What are the causes of metabolic acidosis with a *normal* anion gap?

Conditions causing HCO_3^- loss:
Bowel ischaemia (important cause!)
Diarrhoea
Pancreatic fistula
Addison's disease
Acetazolamide (a diuretic)
Renal tubular acidosis.

What are the causes of metabolic acidosis with $\uparrow$ anionic gap?

Conditions causing $\uparrow$ H^+ (fixed/ organic acids):
mnemonic: **MUD PIES**
Methanol ingestion
Uraemia (renal failure)
Diabetes mellitus (type 1; **ketoacidosis**)
Perfusion deficit (shock causing tissue hypoxia; **lactic acidosis**)
Infection (usually severe; **lactic acidosis**)
Ethylene glycol (antifreeze) ingestion
Salicylates (eg aspirin overdose).

METABOLIC ALKALOSIS

What are the changes?

$\uparrow$**pH, $\uparrow$HCO$_3^-$**

What are the causes?

Conditions causing H^+ loss or HCO_3^- rise. Can be expressed by the equation:

$$\downarrow \text{H}^+ + \text{HCO}_3^- \leftarrow \text{H}_2\text{CO}_3 \leftarrow \text{H}_2\text{O} + \text{CO}_2$$

(loss of H^+ causes a left shift in the equation).

Causes include:
Vomiting (loss of gastric H^+)
Burns
K^+-losing diuretics (via K^+/H^+ co-transport pump)
Bicarbonate ingestion.

RESPIRATORY ACIDOSIS

What are the changes?	$\downarrow$pH, $\uparrow\text{CO}_2$ (O_2 may also be low)
What are the causes?	Conditions causing CO_2 retention, ie any cause of respiratory failure: Chest trauma Pneumonia COPD Diaphragmatic splinting (as in gross bowel obstruction) Myasthaenia gravis (respiratory muscle paralysis).

RESPIRATORY ALKALOSIS

What are the changes?	$\uparrow$pH, $\downarrow\text{CO}_2$ (O_2 may also be high)
What are the causes?	Conditions causing excess blow-off of CO_2, ie any cause of hyperventilation:

CNS causes:
Stroke
Subarachnoid haemorrhage
Meningitis.
Other:
Anxiety
Fever
Altitude.

COMPENSATION

What is compensation?

The body's attempt to return abnormal acid–base status towards the normal. This is seen if in the face of the 1ry abnormality, the pH is normal.

How is this achieved?

In 2 ways: *either* by changes in respiratory rate *or* by changes in renal regulation of H and HCO_3. Metabolic abnormalities invoke respiratory changes, and vice versa:

Metabolic acidosis: ↓pH, ↓HCO_3^-
Compensation: hyperventilation to ↓CO_2

Metabolic alkalosis: ↑pH, ↑HCO_3^-
Compensation: ↓ resp. rate to retain CO_2

Respiratory acidosis: ↓pH, ↑CO_2
Compensation: ↑renal HCO_3^- retention and H^+ excretion

Respiratory alkalosis: ↑pH, ↓CO_2
Compensation: ↑renal HCO_3^- excretion and H^+ retention.

Which one occurs faster?

Respiratory compensation is faster than metabolic compensation, but less efficient.

CHAPTER 5: SURGICAL NUTRITION

What are the daily nutritional requirements in health?

25 kcal/kg (1800 kcal for 70 kg man) 100 g glucose (the brain can only metabolise glucose or ketones) 0.15 g nitrogen/kg or 0.8 g protein/kg.

What are the calorie contents of the main metabolites?

Fats: 9 kcal/g; protein: 4 kcal/g; carbohydrate: 4 kcal/g.

How is a patient's nutritional status assessed?

Clinically: observation (obvious muscle wasting or cachexia); Body Mass Index (BMI)
Anthropometrically: triceps skin fold (use callipers); mid-arm circumference; hand grip
Blood investigations: ↓albumin, prealbumin, transferrin and lymphocyte count.

Which is the best assessment?

Clinical!

How is BMI calculated?

Weight in kg ÷ height in m^2

How much recent weight loss is considered to be risky for surgery?

>10% of original body weight.

What is a patient's nitrogen balance?

A ratio of how much nitrogen a patient is excreting or incorporating into protein.
Positive nitrogen balance: more nitrogen is being incorporated into protein than is being excreted.
Negative nitrogen balance: more nitrogen is being excreted than is being incorporated into muscle.

What is the goal of nutritional support in the surgical patient?

Positive nitrogen balance.

How is nitrogen balance calculated?	[Total protein intake (g) $\div$ 6.25] – [UUN + 4 g] Where: 6.25 = 6.25 g of protein/1 g nitrogen UUN = urine urea nitrogen (grams of nitrogen excreted in urine over 24 h) 4 = 4 g nitrogen lost as insensible losses through GIT and skin.
What is the recommended protein intake in the surgical patient to maintain a positive nitrogen balance?	1.5 g protein/kg/day (as opposed to 0.8 g in the normal adult).
What routes of nutrition do you know of?	**Enteral** and **parenteral**. Of enteral nutrition, the following routes are used: • Oral • Fine-bore NGT (**nasoenteric**) • Tube enterostomy (eg jejunostomy; see Chapter 3, stoma section) • Continuous rectal infusion (**proctoclysis**; rare).
Which route is most preferred?	*Enteral wherever possible!*

What are the indications for parenteral nutrition?	1. Neurological disease:
	  a. Coma
	  b. Intracranial surgery
	  c. CNS trauma
	2. Maxillofacial or neck trauma (swallowing not feasible)
	3. Malfunctioning GIT:
	  a. Fistulae
	  b. Crohn's disease
	  c. Massive small bowel resection (short bowel syndrome)
	  d. Upper GI disease (eg stomach CA, achalasia)
	4. Hypercatabolic state (negative **nitrogen balance**):
	  a. Fever >38°C

b. Severe polytrauma

c. Extensive burns.

How is parenteral nutrition administered?

Via a central line (see Chapter 3).

What are the complications?

Same as for central line (see Chapter 3), but also **electrolyte** and **metabolite imbalances:**

- ↑glucose and risk of HONK
- ↓K, ↑Cl and risk of metabolic acidosis
- ↓Mg, ↓PO_4
- ↓essential fatty acids
- mild **azotaemia** (↑blood urea)
- jaundice.

What is refeeding syndrome?

↓K, Mg and PO_4 in a patient who has been refed after a period of starvation.

What are the metabolic responses to injury, surgery or illness?

Increased metabolic rate (requires more calories) adrenaline, noradrenaline, cortisol, glucagon and growth hormone release, tissue insulin resistance and glucose intolerance, preferential use of lipid as energy source, increased gluconeogenesis, and muscle breakdown.

When should enteric feeding begin on a patient following laparotomy?

Once the patient has begun passing flatus.

What are the fat-soluble vitamins?

Vitamins A, D, E and K

Where are they absorbed?

Terminal ileum.

Which water-soluble vitamin is absorbed in the terminal ileum?

Vitamin B_{12}; dependent on intrinsic factor produced by the parietal cells of the stomach.

What vitamin-deficiency states do you know?   See Table 5.1.

Table 5.1	Alternative name for deficiency	Clinical features
Vitamin A (retinol)	–	Night blindness; xerosis of the conjunctiva and cornea; xerophthalmia and keratomalacia; keratinisation of lung, GI tract, and urinary tract epithelia; increased susceptibility to infections; follicular hyperkeratosis of the skin is common
Vitamin B$_1$ (thiamine)	Beri beri	Irritability, poor memory, sleep disturbances, chest pain, anorexia, abdominal pain, and constipation. CVS symptoms may occur (wet beri beri)
Vitamin B$_6$ (pyridoxine)	–	Dermatosis, glossitis, cheilosis, peripheral neuropathy, and lymphopenia
Vitamin B$_{12}$ (cobalamin)	–	Megaloblastic anaemia; peripheral neuropathy
Vitamin C (ascorbic acid)	Scurvy	Bleeding gums; poor wound healing
Vitamin D (cholecalciferol)	Osteomalacia (adults) Rickets (children)	Bowing of the long bones, short stature in children, and flattening of the pelvic bones, which narrows the pelvic outlet

Which vitamin ↑Fe absorption?   Vitamin C.

Which mineral is important in wound healing?   Zinc.

CHAPTER 6: POST-OPERATIVE COMPLICATIONS

How do you classify post-operative complications?

Local: involving the operation site itself

General: affecting the systems of the body eg respiratory, cardiovascular and gastrointestinal.

or

Immediate: within 24 hours
Early: within 4 weeks
Late: after 4 weeks.

How is post-op haemorrhage classified?

1ry: immediately (occurring at operation)

2ry: reactionary (<24 hours) subsequent to blood pressure rise post-operatively

3ry: (>24 hours) subsequent to **infection**, typically around day 10.

What must you be wary of in the bleeding post-op patient?

Haemorrhagic (hypovolaemic) shock!

What would you do if the blood pressure falls post-operatively?

Assume haemorrhagic shock until proven otherwise! Do the following:
1. Immediately assess airway, breathing and circulation (ABCs)
2. Check the following:
   a. Observations
   b. Capillary refill time
   c. Urine output
3. Take a brief history of the procedure undertaken and examine the following:
   a. General signs of shock (cool, clammy peripheries; tachycardia; ↓JVP)
   b. Operation site for bleeding/ discharge/tenderness/ ecchymoses
   c. Nasogastric aspirate and drain contents and amount; fistulae output

4. Perform the **rule of tubes**! Which of the following tubes does the patient need if not already in place?
   a. Oxygen mask
   b. IV Line with fluids
   c. Urinary catheter
   d. NGT.

What then?

Maintain systolic BP above 90 mmHg, replacing fluid like for like (ie for whatever amount of fluid has been lost, replace with a similar amount of fluid).

How is this best done?

By giving IV **colloid**, initially in boluses of 100 ml under close observation. Colloids (eg Gelofusin) are macromolecular and so remain in and expand the circulating volume for longer when compared with crystalloids (eg normal saline).

What are potential bleeding sites?

1. Ruptured clot
2. Misplaced sutures
3. Ischaemic bowel (in GI surgery)
4. Wound
5. Drain site.

Besides bleeding, what other causes of post-op hypotension do you know of?

Cardiac insult: eg myocardial infarction:
Order: ECG (ST changes), blood investigations including cardiac enzymes, and CXR.
Prescribe: oxygen, aspirin, GTN, and diamorphine
Inform: cardiologist, ITU.
Pulmonary insult: eg pulmonary embolism:
Order: ECG ($S_1Q_3T_3$ changes), blood investigations including D-dimer and ABGs, CXR (pulmonary wedge)
Prescribe: oxygen and heparin or low molecular-weight heparins (LMWHs)

Inform: respiratory team, ITU.

Infectious insult: eg septicaemia:
Order: blood investigations including blood cultures, ECG, CXR (r/o pneumonia)
Prescribe: best-guess antibiotics targeting the most likely source or broad spectrum antibiotics, until culture results return
Inform: microbiologist, on-call physician, ITU.

Neurogenic insult: eg epidural anaesthesia (decreases sympathetic drive, causing vasodilatation and hypotension):
Inform: anaesthetist.

In *all* cases, begin with ABCs and follow on as with haemorrhagic shock as before. *Only then* can individual treatments begin!

What are the causes of pulmonary embolism?

mnemonic: **TOM SCHREPFER**
Trauma
Obesity
Malignancy (a hypercoagulable state)
Surgery (esp. orthopaedic and pelvic)
Cardiac disease
Hospitalisation (prolonged)
Rest (bed-ridden patients)
Elderly
Past history of DVT/**P**E/**P**regnancy
Fracture (esp. of long bones)
o**E**strogen (OCP, HRT)
Road trip (eg long flight).

Why would the blood pressure *rise* post operatively?

Pain is the most common reason. Causes include:
1. Inadequate analgesia
2. Urinary retention
3. Anxiety
Known pre-operative hypertension (check their medication!).

What are the causes of post-op pyrexia?

mnemonic: **8 Cs**
Catheter (urinary tract infection [UTI])
Cannula/**C**entral Line (phlebitis or drug allergy)
Cut (wound infection; map out the limits of any spreading **C**ellulitis with a pen for daily follow-up purposes post-antibiotics)
Chest (atelectasis or PE)
Calf (DVT [days 7–10])
Collection (of pus, eg pelvic, subphrenic).

Can the cause of pyrexia be assumed by the amount of days post-op?

Generally, yes (but not a hard and fast rule!):
1st 24 hours: systemic response to surgery (physiological)
Days 1–3: atelectasis, pneumonia
Days 4–7: wound infection, UTI, intra-abdominal sepsis (collection, etc), anastomotic dehiscence
Days 7–10: DVT, PE.

What are the standard investigations for post-op pyrexia?

Blood investigations:
1. FBC
2. U+Es
3. CRP
4. Blood cultures
5. ABGs
6. D-dimers (if PE suspected).
Other investigations:
1. Wound swabs and body fluids (urine, drain specimens, sputum) for microscopy, culture and sensitivity
2. If the chest is involved, order CXR and venous Doppler USS of the calves.

What is the management?

1. Oxygen
2. Fluids
3. Intravenous cefuroxime with metronidazole or co-amoxiclav are

recognized regimens for 5 days pending culture results, and discontinue if infection is absent.
4. Treat underlying cause once identified.

What are the causes of post-op confusion?

mnemonic: **DELIRIUM**
Drugs
Electrolyte imbalance
Lack of drugs (alcohol/heroin withdrawal)
Infection/sepsis
Reduced sensory input (new surroundings, blindness)
Intracranial problems (TIA, stroke, post-ictal state)
Urinary retention
Myocardial problems (infarction, arrhythmias).

What specific complications can occur post-abdominal surgery?

1. Intra-abdominal bleeding
2. Anastomotic dehiscence (day 4–7)
3. Bowel ischaemia
4. Wound dehiscence (day 4–5)
5. Burst abdomen (day 10)
6. Bowel obstruction (functional or mechanical).

What are the warning signs?

1. Pyrexia
2. Pain
3. Peritonism
4. Pink serous fluid discharge (burst abdomen)
5. Abdominal haematoma
6. Obstipation with tinkling bowel sounds (mechanical obstruction; see Chapter 18).

Which patients are at risk for post-op renal failure?

mnemonic: **LORD help these patients!**

Liver disease (esp. obstructive jaundice)

Obstructive nephropathy (ie post-renal failure 2ry to urinary retention, eg post-prostatectomy clot, UTI)/**O**ld people

Renal vascular disease (diabetic nephropathy, atherosclerotic renal disease)

Drugs (NSAIDs, ACE inhibitors).

What is adult respiratory distress syndrome (ARDS)?

Non-cardiogenic pulmonary oedema with a normal pulmonary capillary wedge pressure (PCWP) (ie pulmonary oedema not caused by CCF). It is precipitated by various acute processes that directly or indirectly injure the lung. It is characterised by:
1. Stiff lungs
2. Refractory hypoxaemia ($PaO_2/FiO_2 < 200$)
3. Diffuse, patchy infiltrates on CXR
4. Mortality of approximately 50%.

So what *is* PCWP?

It is an estimate of the end-diastolic volume (EDV) of the heart, and hence an estimate of **preload**. EDV (and preload) is $\uparrow$ in CCF as contractility is reduced and less blood is pumped out per contraction. In ARDS, PCWP is normal (defining point!).

How is PCWP measured?

Via cardiac catheterisation. Normal range is 5–13 mmHg.

What are the causes of ARDS?

mnemonic: **BEAT ARDS**
Blood transfusion (massive)/**B**urns
Embolism (fat, air or amniotic fluid)
Aspiration
Trauma (polytrauma, direct chest trauma)
Acute pancreatitis
Radiation (eg post-radiotherapy)
DIC/**D**rug overdose/near-**D**rowning/**D**ialysis/
Diffuse pneumonia (viral, fungal or bacterial)
Sepsis/**S**hock/**S**moke inhalation.

How do you manage ARDS?

mnemonic: **ARDS!**
Avoid causes of pulmonary oedema (CCF, pneumonia, etc)
Respiratory assistance:
- Mechanical ventilation
- PEEP
- IRV (encourages alveolar recruitment)
- Inhaled nitrous oxide (improves V/Q quotient)

Dependent body positions (gravity ↑ lung blood flow)
Secretions (avoid with help of physiotherapist).

CHAPTER 7: ANAESTHESIA

PRE-OPERATIVE ASSESSMENT

How does the physical status of a patient relate to mortality?

Based on the American Society of Anaesthesiologists (ASA) rating scale (see Table 7.1)

Table 7.1

ASA rating	Mortality risk
I. Normal healthy patient	0.05%
II. Mild systemic disease	0.4%
III. Severe systemic disease limiting activity but not incapacitating	4.5%
IV. Incapacitating systemic disease that is a constant threat to life	25%
V. Moribund, not expected to survive with or without the operation	50%
Add E for emergency operation	

What factors predict a difficult intubation?

Several tests can be used. Accuracy is improved by combining the results from more than one:

Thyromental distance: from prominence of thyroid cartilage to bony point on chin with the neck fully extended. Distance of less than 7 cm suggests difficult intubation.

Wilson score: comprises evaluation of 5 factors:
1. Weight
2. Receding mandible
3. Degree of head and neck movement
4. Degree of jaw movement
5. Buck teeth.

Mallampati grading: an estimate of the size of the tongue in the pharynx.

Assessed as the anaesthetist sits opposite the patient and asks them to open their mouth as wide as they can. The view obtained correlates to: *Grade:*
1. Faucial pillars, soft palate, uvula
2. Faucial pillars, soft palate, uvula masked by tongue
3. Only soft palate visible
4. Soft palate not visible.

What are pre-medications?

Any drug administered in the period prior to induction of anaesthesia.
mnemonic: remember the **6 As:**
1. **A**nxiolytics: usually benzodiazepines
2. **A**mnesics
3. **A**nalgesics
4. **A**ntacids: reduce gastric acid load
5. **A**nti-autonomics: to prevent vagally mediated bradycardias and reduce secretions
6. **A**ntiemetics: dopamine or histamine antagonists commonly.

CARDIOVASCULAR

How can cardiovascular risk be assessed pre-operatively?

By the following:
Clinical Risk: major predictors
- Recent MI (within 30 days)
- Unstable or severe angina
- Decompensated CCF
- Severe valvular disease
- Significant arrhythmia:
  1. High grade AV block
  2. Symptomatic ventricular arrhythmia
  3. Uncontrolled rate of supraventricular arrhythmia.

Functional Risk: poor functional capacity is associated with increasing cardiovascular complications. Assess the patient's functional capacity: activities of daily living, walking distance, ability to climb stairs, jogging, sports, etc.

Surgical Risk:
- *High:* emergency, aortic, peripheral vascular, prolonged operations with large fluid shifts
- *Intermediate:* orthopaedic, urologic, uncomplicated abdominal, head and neck, thoracic surgery
- *Low:* endoscopic, breast, cataract surgery.

Which tests would you do in a patient with cardiovascular disease?

Blood investigations:
1. FBC: anaemia can worsen ischaemia
2. U&Es: reno-vascular disease
3. Blood sugar: diabetes (controlled?)

Bedside tests:
1. Urine dipstick
2. ECG: mandatory

Imaging:
1. CXR: if no X-ray within 12 months, or positive clinical examination (eg crepitations in CCF)
2. Echocardiogram: for investigation of valvular disease; **dobutamine stress echo** may be useful for further assessment of those considered at intermediate cardiovascular risk
3. Dipyridamole-thallium imaging: for further stratification of those considered at intermediate cardiovascular risk.

Other tests:
1. 24 h tape: suspected dysrhythmias

2. Exercise tolerance test/interventional cardiology as deemed necessary by cardiologist.

RESPIRATORY

What post-operative problems are important when considering a patient with respiratory disease?

Patients with respiratory disease (eg COPD, asthma, restrictive lung disease) are more prone to post-op respiratory tract infections. The risks are greater if the patient is obese or undergoing thoracic/upper abdominal surgery where:

- Hypoventilation may lead to **basal atelectasis** ($\downarrow$ functional residual capacity by 20–60%)
- Pain may prevent expectoration, deep inhalation, and mobilisation. Resultant sputum retention may lead to mucus plugging and lung collapse or act as a nidus for infection.

How could you optimise a patient with respiratory disease?

By doing the following:
Pre-operative measures:
1. Maximise bronchodilator therapy (eg salbutamol)
2. Control infection
3. Smoking cessation
4. Weight loss if obese
5. Physiotherapy (eg incentive spirometry, postural drainage)
6. Drain pleural effusions
7. Minimise oxygen requirements.
Post-operative measures:
1. Physiotherapy and mobilisation
2. DVT prophylaxis
3. Optimise analgesia
4. Elective HDU admission.

Which tests would you do in a patient with respiratory disease?

Blood investigations:
1. FBC: infection, polycythaemia
2. U&Es
3. ABG: type I/II respiratory failure.

Bedside tests:
1. Peak flow
2. Urine dipstick
3. ECG: cor pulmonale (right axis deviation), right ventricular hypertrophy (tall QRS complexes in V1, V2).

Imaging: CXR to r/o the following:
1. Acute respiratory symptoms
2. Chronic disease without CXR last 12 months
3. Suspected TB/malignancy.

Other tests:
1. V/Q scan: to estimate differential pulmonary performance prior to thoracic surgery (eg lobectomy/pneumonectomy)
2. Spirometry: to assess lung function and capacities.

METABOLIC

What factors are important when considering a patient with liver disease?

Keep the following in mind:
1. Abnormal drug handling:
   a. Drugs that undergo hepatic metabolisation may accumulate
   b. Pt. more sensitive to opioids and sedatives: may provoke encephalopathy
2. Metabolic disturbance: monitor U&Es; beware **hepatorenal syndrome** (acute kidney failure occurring without other cause in a person with severe liver disease)
3. Abnormal clotting: monitor INR, APTT

4. Complications of cirrhosis: varices, ascites, encephalopathy
5. Infection risk
6. Poor nutritional state
7. **Secondary hyperaldosteronism**: occurs due to low albumin production by the liver, and hence ↓ intravascular oncotic pressure. ↑ Aldosterone production by adrenals occurs in an attempt to maintain blood pressure. Take care with saline infusions (↑ aldosterone already causing salt retention; risk of hypernatraemia).

And patients with renal failure?

Renal failure:
1. Abnormal renal excretion of drugs:
    a. alter the dosage of renally excreted drugs depending upon GFR
    b. avoid nephrotoxins eg gentamicin, NSAIDS
2. Metabolic disturbance: beware acute on chronic renal failure
3. Careful fluid balance: easily overloaded
4. Complications of chronic renal failure: IHD, anaemia, hypertension, bone disease, bleeding tendency
5. Infection risk.

What options are there for glycaemic control in the diabetic patient undergoing surgery?

General:
1. Optimise glycaemic control in the run up to surgery. Involve GP as necessary
2. Try to put diabetic patients first on the operating list so avoiding complications with prolonged fasting.

Insulin dependent (Type 1) diabetics:

1. Stop all long acting insulin the night before surgery
2. Omit morning s/c insulin and switch to IV insulin according to sliding scale. Some units advocate a dextrose/potassium/insulin (GKI) regime with 500 ml bags of 5–10% dextrose, 10 mmol KCl, and a variable amount of insulin adjusted 4 hourly according to BM. The rationale is provision of basal insulin, suppression of ketone production, and avoidance of possible complications (eg hypoglycaemia) if monitoring is sub-optimal
3. Monitor BM regularly aiming for normoglycaemia during surgery
4. Switch to regular s/c insulin only after the patient takes their second meal.

Non-insulin dependent (Type 2) diabetics:

1. If fasting BM >15 on the morning of surgery treat as for type 1
2. Halve dose of long-acting sulphonylurea the day prior to surgery
3. Omit morning dose on the day of surgery
4. If major operation (especially GI) where the patient may not be eating for several days, switch to IV insulin sliding scale.

ANAESTHESIA AND ANALGESIA

ANAESTHESIA

What are the aims of surgical anaesthesia?

mnemonic: The **five As**:
1. **A**naesthesia
2. **A**nalgesia
3. **A**reflexia
4. **A**mnesia
5. **A**utonomic stability.

These aims are not adequately met by using a single agent hence the combined use of premeds, anaesthetic agents, muscle relaxants, analgesics to produce **'balanced' anaesthesia**.

What are the properties of the ideal anaesthetic agent?

Physical:
1. Non-flammable, non-explosive at room temperature
2. Stable in light
3. Long half life
4. Easily stored
5. Cheap.

Biological:
1. Pleasant to inhale/painless to inject
2. Fast onset
3. High potency
4. Minimal systemic effects
5. Non-toxic to theatre personnel.

What was the first anaesthetic agent used?

Ether was the first agent used to induce surgical anaesthesia. It is little used nowadays except in developing countries owing to its flammability and side-effects.

What are the properties of the anaesthetic drugs in common use?

Intravenous (induction) agents: normally **some** produce their effect in one arm–brain circulation time, hence contra-indicated if the anaesthetist is not confident of being able to maintain the airway:

Propofol:

- Suitable for induction and maintenance of anaesthesia
- Provides rapid induction and recovery without hangover (4–7 min)
- Causes hypotension secondary to bradycardia and vasodilatation.

Etomidate:

- Provides rapid induction and recovery without hangover
- Cannot be used for maintenance of anaesthesia as prolonged use suppresses adrenocortical function
- Less cardiovascular side effects than other IV agents.

Thiopentone: short-acting barbiturate that accumulates after repeated doses, hence not used for maintenance.

Ketamine:

- Slower onset of induction and recovery than other IV agents
- Rarely used now owing to troublesome hallucinations and other psychotic symptoms
- Minimal cardiovascular or respiratory depression, hence useful in emergency surgery with unstable patients.

Inhalation agents: can be used for induction (slower than IV agents) and maintenance of anaesthesia:

Nitrous oxide (NO):

- A non-irritant, sweet smelling gas
- A good analgesic but poor anaesthetic, it is usually administered in a 70/30 ratio with oxygen to provide analgesia

accompanying other inhalational anaesthetic agents
- Concomitant use of NO decreases the necessary dose of other inhaled anaesthetics by up to 50%.

Halothane:
- A volatile liquid
- Repeat doses may cause 'halothane hepatitis'
- Risk of malignant hyperpyrexia
- Arrhythmias.

Halogenated ether derivatives:
eg isoflurane, sevoflurane
- Volatile liquids with varying potencies
- All cause hypotension and ventilatory depression
- Lower incidence of malignant hyperpyrexia than with halothane.

How is GA induced?

GA (general anaesthetic) is commonly induced with an IV anaesthetic agent that causes a rapid loss of consciousness and subsequently maintained with inhalation agents.

What is TIVA?

Total **I**ntra**V**enous **A**naesthesia: IV anaesthetic agents are used for induction and maintenance with supplementary IV muscle relaxants and analgesia. The benefits of TIVA are:
- Less risk of malignant hyperpyrexia and hepatitis
- Less risk of adverse reactions as fewer drugs are used
- Better control of depth of anaesthesia.

What types of muscle relaxants do you know of?

Depolarising and non-depolarising.

What is the main depolarizing muscle relaxant used?	Suxamethonium.
How does it work?	It mimics the action of acetylcholine at the neuromuscular junction, causing depolarisation. Unlike acetylcholine however it is not hydrolysed by acetylcholinesterases but undergoes slower metabolisation by plasma pseudo-cholinesterases. The result is a prolonged neuromuscular block resulting in paralysis.
What is its advantage?	Suxemethonium has a rapid onset and short duration of action making it ideal for facilitating intubation, especially in **crash induction** where intubation is an emergency.
What are its risks?	In patients deficient in pseudo-cholinesterases, there may be a delayed recovery. It can also cause **hyperkalaemia**.
Give examples of non-depolarising muscle relaxants	Atracurium, pancuronium, vercuronium.
How do non-depolarising agents work?	Compete with acetylcholine for receptor sites at the motor end plate but do not cause depolarisation. Their action may be reversed with anticholinesterases such as neostigmine.
What is their advantage?	They have a slower onset but their longer duration of action than suxamethonium makes them more suitable for longer operations.
What is malignant hyperpyrexia?	A condition characterised by the development of masseter or generalised skeletal muscle rigidity, rising body temperature, acidosis,

hypoxia, and rhabdomyolysis caused by a defect in the sarcoplasmic reticulum calcium release channel, or ryanodine receptor (RYR1) that results in altered calcium homeostasis. It has a 30% mortality.

Which drugs are the major culprits?

Halothane and suxamethonium account for 80% of cases.

How is it treated?

By the following:
1. Stop the precipitant
2. High flow oxygen
3. External cooling
4. ABG for acidosis, send bloods for U+Es and CK
5. Dantrolene (calcium antagonist) IV 1–2.5 mg/kg every 10 min up to a maximum 10 mg/kg
6. Cooled IV fluids for hypotension
7. Procainamide to prevent ventricular dysrythmias
8. Seizures are common; have anti-convulsants to hand.

ANALGESIA

Why is analgesia important post-operatively?

Pain has multi-system effects:
Cardiovascular: increased myocardial oxygen requirements
Respiratory: reduced cough, sputum retention, atelectasis, infection
Gastrointestinal: constipation, reduced gastric emptying
Genitourinary: urinary retention
Endocrine: protein consumption, hyperglycaemia
Musculoskeletal: immobility, pressure sores, DVTs
Neurological: insomnia, fatigue, anxiety, neuroendocrine stress response, ADH release.

What modalities of analgesia are available?

Psychological:
1. Explanation and education
2. Relaxation
3. Hypnosis.

Physical:
1. Physiotherapy
2. Wound splinting
3. Transcutaneous Electric Nerve Stimulation (TENS)
4. Cold or heat
5. Acupuncture.

Pharmacological:
1. Simple analgesia
2. Opiates
3. Local and regional anaesthetics.

What routes are available for administration of analgesia?

See Table 7.2.

Table 7.2

Route	Advantages	Disadvantages
Oral	Acceptability Self administration	Delayed absorption 1st pass metabolism
Sublingual	Rapid absorption Avoids 1st pass metabolism	Few available preparations Inconvenient
Rectal	Rapid absorption Smaller doses Avoids 1st pass metabolism	Unacceptability Few available preparations Erratic absorption
Transdermal	Convenient Sustained release	Erratic absorption
Subcutaneous	Continuous infusions	Irritation Accumulation
Intramuscular	Sustained release	Painful Erratic bioavailability
Intravenous	Rapid effect	Peaks and troughs Toxicity-overdose
Epidural/spinal	Can produce surgical analgesia	Technical Overdose problematic

What is Patient Controlled Analgesia (PCA)?

The patient is able to self-administer a small bolus of IV opioid analgesia via a demand button. A preset background infusion of opiate may be concurrently infused if severe pain is anticipated.

Advantages:
- Better titration of analgesia to pain, with in theory a more constant plasma concentration of analgesic and fewer peaks and troughs
- Patient feels in control.

Disadvantages:
- Technical to institute
- Requires able patient ie conscious, able to press button (eg rheumatoid arthritis)
- Potential for overdose if incorrectly setup.

How is overdose prevented?

By capping the maximal bolus and infusion dose, and ensuring an adequate 'lock-out' period after each bolus.

What are the complications of opiates?

The following:
CNS: analgesia, respiratory depression, sedation, euphoria, dependence, nausea, pupil constriction
Respiratory: apnoea, anti-tussive, bronchospasm
Gastrointestinal: delayed gastric emptying, constipation, biliary spasm
Cardiovascular: bradycardia, vasodilatation, hypotension
Genitourinary: urinary retention
Skin: pruritis
Endocrine: ADH and catecholamine release.

How would you manage an opiate overdose?	1. Stop opiates
	2. High flow oxygen
	3. If the patient is apnoeic, commence bag-mask valve ventilation with airway control
	4. Naloxone (pure opioid antagonist) IV 0.2–0.4 mg at 3 minute intervals up to 2 mg max. Naloxone has a short half-life and an infusion may be necessary to avoid resedation. Complete reversal of opiate action is often unnecessary and will lead to reversal of analgesia. Naloxone may precipitate withdrawal in the opiate dependent patient.

SURGICAL ITU

CARDIOVASCULAR SYSTEM

What are the important CVS formulae?	Cardiac output = heart rate × stroke volume Mean arterial pressure = $[(2 \times \text{diastolic}) + \text{systolic}]/3$
What is shock?	A state of cardiovascular collapse resulting in inadequate tissue perfusion and end organ dysfunction. Hypotension and tachycardia may or may not be present (see Chapter 11).
What are the aims of management in shock in ITU?	Following initial resuscitation, the priorities in shock are: • Correction of underlying cause: shock is a syndrome and not a diagnosis • Optimise oxygen delivery: – Optimise cardiac output (CO = HR × SV) – Optimise haemoglobin: 8–10 g/dl

- Maximise oxygen saturations
- Optimise organ perfusion
- Support for organ failure.

Goals of treatment are often directed at values of:

- Mean arterial pressure >65 mmHg
- Central venous pressure 8–12 mmHg
- Urine output >0.5 ml/kg/h
- Central venous saturations >70%

How is CO optimised?   Adequate fluid resuscitation.

And if this fails?   If CO remains inadequate despite optimised fluid resuscitation, **inotropic support** may be initiated to improve cardiac contractility and performance.

What inotropes do you know?   See Table 7.3.

Table 7.3

Inotrope	Receptors	Actions	Classification
Epinephrine (adrenaline)	α_1, β_1, β_2	Increase heart rate and stroke volume Vasoconstriction	Inopressor
Dobutamine	β_2, DA	Increase heart rate and stroke volume Vasodilator	Inodilator
Dopamine	DA, α_1, β_1, β_2	*Low dose: <5 µg/kg/min* Renal, mesenteric artery dilatation *Intermediate dose: 5–10 µg/kg/min* Increase heart rate and stroke volume *High dose: >10 µg/kg/min* Increase heart rate and stroke volume Vasoconstriction	Inodilator Inopressor

How is organ perfusion optimised?

By optimising the **perfusion pressure** (afterload). This, in turn, is dependent on blood pressure.

How is perfusion pressure optimised?

Maintaining adequate volume status and CO.

And if this fails?

If blood pressure remains low despite adequate volume status and cardiac output, **vasopressors** may be used to increase **systemic vascular resistance** and raise blood pressure in order to perfuse vital organs. (Vasopressors have no appreciable direct effect on CO.)

What should be monitored when using vasopressors?

Vasopressor therapy should be titrated against the patients mean arterial blood pressure (MAP) and reduced wherever possible to avoid adverse effects.

What vasopressors do you know of?

See Table 7.4.

Table 7.4

Vasopressor	Receptor	Actions	Classification
Norepinephrine (noradrenaline)	α_1	Peripheral vasoconstriction	Vasopressor
Phenylephrine	α_1	Peripheral vasoconstriction	Vasopressor

How is the response to inotropic/vasopressor support monitored?

Clinical examination and bedside tests:

1. Neurological status: GCS (adequate cerebral perfusion)
2. Skin temperature and colour
3. Peripheral perfusion and capillary refill
4. Pulse: rate and character analysis
5. Blood pressure, pulse pressure
6. Urine output (adequate renal perfusion).

Invasive monitoring:

1. Arterial line: beat to beat blood pressure and waveform analysis
2. CVP with dynamic assessment after fluid challenges
3. Pulmonary artery catheterisation: estimates pulmonary capillary wedge pressure (PCWP) a surrogate for left ventricular filling pressures
4. Pulse contour analysis: allows calculation of cardiac output, stroke volume, systemic vascular resistance
5. Oesophageal Doppler: can estimate cardiac output and stroke volume by cross-sectional analysis of flow through the aorta.

RESPIRATORY SYSTEM

How is respiratory failure defined?

On blood gas analysis:

Type I (hypoxaemic):

$PaO_2 < 8$ kpa, $PaCO_2 < 6$ kpa. Represents ventilation perfusion mismatch (V/Q), a function of dead space ventilation and shunt.

Causes:

- Asthma
- COPD
- Pulmonary embolus
- Pulmonary oedema
- Pneumonia
- Adult Respiratory Distress Syndrome (ARDS).

Type II (hypercapnic):

$PaO_2 < 8$ kpa, $PaCO_2 > 6$ kpa. Represents hypoventilation with or without a degree of V/Q mismatch.

Causes:

- *Pulmonary disease:* COPD, asthma, pneumonia

- *Neuromuscular disease:* spinal cord injury, phrenic nerve injury, myasthenia gravis
- *Chest wall abnormality:* kyphoscoliosis, trauma
- *Reduced respiratory drive:* sedatives, CVA/brain injury.

What is the alveolar–arterial gradient?

Estimates the difference between the partial pressure of alveolar and arterial oxygen. A large difference suggests more severe disease. (It can be approximated by: $F_iO_2\%-PaCO_2-PaO_2$.)

What is CPAP?

Continuous **P**ositive **A**irway **P**ressure: a form of respiratory support for spontaneously breathing patients that provides a constant positive pressure throughout the airway cycle.

How is it given?

Either by application of a tight fitting face mask or via an endotracheal/tracheostomy tube.

How does it work?

It works by:
- Splinting open the airways thus recruiting collapsed lung, increasing the functional residual capacity (FRC)
- Increased FRC improves oxygenation and lung compliance.

What are the indications for CPAP?

CPAP requires a conscious, tolerant patient who is able to maintain their own airway and initiate respiration. It can be used for:
- Treatment of acute respiratory failure where face mask oxygen is insufficient and intubation not yet necessary or inappropriate
- Ventilator weaning
- Obstructive sleep apnoea (OSA).

What are the complications of CPAP?

1. Cardiovascular compromise: raised intra-thoracic pressure decreases venous return
2. Gastric distension and risk of aspiration
3. Nasal bridge skin pressure necrosis
4. Drying of the airway
5. Pneumothorax.

What are the indications for intubation and mechanical ventilation?

mnemonic: **3A 4H**
Airway protection: GCS < 8
Airway toilet and secretion control
Apnoeic patient
Head injury for control of $PaCO_2$ (aiming for normocapnoea)
Hypoxaemia PaO_2 < 8 kpa
Hypoventilation with hypercapnoea and acidosis
Hyperventilation (RR > 35) with impending exhaustion.

A **tracheostomy** should be contemplated in all patients expected to be intubated for >7 days.

RENAL

What are the indications for Renal Replacement Therapy (RRT)?

1. Hyperkalaemia: K > 6.5
2. Acidosis pH < 7.1
3. Fluid overload: refractory pulmonary oedema
4. Symptomatic uraemia: usually urea > 40 mmol/L but may be lower in acute presentations
5. Removal of toxic metabolites.

How is RRT given?

Peritoneal dialysis (PD): fluid exchange via catheter inserted into peritoneal cavity. Rarely used in the ITU setting as it is less effective at clearing solutes than other modes of RRT and the increased intra-abdominal volume may splint the diaphragm leading to respiratory difficulties. Contra-indicated in abdominal pathology.

Intermittent haemodialysis (IHD): fast and effective method for RRT, done via a surgically created arterio-venous (A-V) shunt. The main problem is that the large fluid shifts may not be tolerated by haemodynamically unstable patients.

Continuous renal replacement (CRRT): can be VenoVenous (VV) or ArterioVenous (AV), and utilise either:
- HaemoFiltration (CAVH/CVVH)
- HaemoDialysis (CAVHD/CVVHD)
- HaemoDiaFiltration (CAVHDF/ CVVHDF).

CRRT has slower flow rates than IHD and is often tolerated by patients too unstable for intermittent haemodialysis.

Where is CRRT particularly useful?

1. **Raised intracranial pressure:** slower solute transfer makes it useful for these patients where rapid changes in osmolarity may be dangerous.
2. **Sepsis:** where the clearance of inflammatory mediators may be beneficial.

SEPTICAEMIA

What is sepsis?

Can be classified as a diagnosis of infection in the presence of 2 of the 4 signs of the **Systemic Inflammatory Response Syndrome (SIRS)**:
1. Temperature < 36 or > 38.3°C
2. WCC < 4 or > 12

3. Heart Rate > 100
4. Respiratory rate > 20.
Severe sepsis: SIRS + any evidence of end organ dysfunction.
Septic shock: SIRS + hypotension refractory to volume replacement.

What is the management?

The following:
1. Early fluid resuscitation with 6 h goal directed targets:
   - MAP > 65 mmHg
   - CVP 8–12 mmHg
   - Urine output > 0.5 ml/kg/h
   - Central venous saturations ($ScVO_2$) > 70%
   - Monitor lactate for response, <2 mmol/L ideal.

   If unable to reach targets despite adequate fluid resuscitation, commence inotropes or vasopressors. Maintain Hb 7–9 g/dL.
2. Take 2× blood cultures before commencing appropriate broad spectrum antibiotics
3. Control source of infection, initiate full septic screen, narrow antibiotic spectrum once organisms and sensitivities acquired
4. Ventilate with lung protective strategies
5. Tight glycaemic control BM < 8.3
6. Commence steroids after short synacthen test if on vasopressors or adrenal insufficiency suspected
7. Consider Activated Protein C (APC)
8. DVT and stress ulcer prophylaxis
9. Target sedation to pre-determined end-points. Avoid neuromuscular blockers if possible

10. Renal replacement therapy as warranted.

(See R Phillip Dellinger, Jean M Carlet et al. Surviving Sepsis Campaign guidelines for management of severe sepsis and septic shock. *Crit Care Med* 2004; 32(3): 858–873.)

CHAPTER 8: MINIMAL ACCESS SURGERY

What is minimal access surgery (MAS)?

Surgery carried out via a minimally invasive procedure using an **endoscope**.

What is it also known as?

Key-hole surgery or band-aid surgery.

What is laparoscopy?

Visualisation of the peritoneal cavity with special endoscopes (known as **laparoscopes**) passed through **ports** in the abdominal wall. A **pneumoperitoneum** is created prior to introduction of the laparoscope.

What is a pneumoperitoneum?

Insufflation of gas into the peritoneal cavity causing the abdominal wall to distend from the abdominal viscera, hence making laparoscopy and MAS technically feasible.

How is it performed?

2 approaches:
Open induction (Hasson):
1. 1–2 cm transverse infra-umbilical incision made through skin, subcutaneous fat, Camper's and Scarpa's facia to the underlying linea alba
2. Linea alba is incised and 2 stay sutures applied, allowing direct vision inside the peritoneal cavity.
3. A finger is inserted to check and remove any adhesions
4. A blunt port is inserted and carbon dioxide gas supply is connected to establish the pneumoperitoneum.
5. Fibreoptic camera is inserted into port and further ports are placed elsewhere in abdominal wall *under direct vision of the camera* with the aid of a fitted, sharp spring-loaded **trocar** (allows penetration through the

abdominal layers without incision beyond the skin; has a plastic guard that projects beyond the sharp point once the peritoneum has been entered).

Closed (blind) induction (Veress needle):

1. A hollow Veress needle (with spring-loaded **obturator** that covers the sharp needle once the peritoneal cavity has been entered) is inserted just below the umbilicus through all layers of the abdomen.
2. Carbon dioxide is attached and pneunoperitoneum is induced. The rest of the steps follow open induction.

How do we know we are in the abdominal cavity rather than in a visceral organ when using closed induction?

There are 2 tests:
Drop test: a drop of saline is dropped into the open Luer fitting of the Verres needle and should fall freely from sight into the peritoneal cavity due to the subatmospheric pressure within.
Saline injection: a small amount of saline is injected into the peritoneal cavity via the Verres needle; it should go freely, and aspiration should draw air back into the syringe, not blood, bile or bowel contents.

How should carbon dioxide be insufflated?

Slowly! The pressure should not rise drastically fast.

Why is carbon dioxide used?

It is an **inert gas**. Residual is absorbed post-procedure.

How may ports in all should be used?

1 for diagnostic laparoscopy and 2 or more for surgical procedures. The operation dictates the anatomical site chosen for further port insertion.

How big should the ports be?

10 mm port for fibreoptic camera, producing a high resolution magnified image; 5 mm port for instruments. (Skin incisions are 10 mm or 5 mm accordingly).

3 mm port is a new size available in certain centres; called mini/micro/needloscopic surgery.

What types of laparoscopes do you know of?

Usually a 10 mm scope (available in 5 mm), field of view being 0° or 30° angles. Usually, 0° is used for a laparoscopic cholecystectomy and 30° for laparoscopic nephrectomy.

What instruments can be used during laparoscopic MAS?

Dissectors, scissors, graspers, staplers and diathermy.

What are the contraindications to laparoscopy/MAS?

Absolute: *mnemonic:* **SCOPE**
Shock (uncontrolled)
Cirrhosis/**C**lotting abnormalities
Obstruction (intestinal)
Peritonitis (generalised)
Ether (failure to tolerate general anaesthetic).

Relative: *mnemonic:* **GAPE**
Gross obesity
Abdominal aortic aneurysm
Pregnancy
Excessive adhesions.

What are the advantages of MAS?

1. No cutting of muscles, as ports are placed between muscle fibres, with early return to normal activity
2. Reduces hospital stay
3. Cosmetic acceptability
4. Reduced pain due to smaller skin incisions
5. Reduced complications of wound infection and post-op chest complications

6. Less risk with co-morbidity (eg diabetes) due to reduced physiological insult
7. Minimal risk of incisional hernias
8. Diagnostic potential.
9. Video records
10. Decreased viral contact eg HIV/Hep B.

What are the disadvantages?

1. No tactile feedback: total reliance on hand-eye coordination
2. Longer procedures
3. High cost of equipment and training (steep learning curve)
4. Possible increased incidence of metastasis at port sites.
5. Some serious and frequent risks (see below).

What are the risks?

Serious:

1. Misplacement of needle with damage to bowel, bladder, major vessels and abdominal wall emphysema
2. Failure to gain entry to abdominal cavity
3. Difficulty in controlling bleeding
4. Carbon dioxide embolus and metabolic acidosis post-pneumoperitoneum
5. Hypotension and reflex tachycardia 2ry to reduced cardiac venous return (side-effect of pneumoperitoneum).

Frequent:

1. Bruising
2. Shoulder tip pain (irritation of peritoneum overlying the diaphragm 2ry to pneumoperitoneum); self-limiting.

Complications rate of diagnostic laparoscopy is 2:1000.

When should MAS be converted to open surgery?

In the following situations:
1. More extensive disease requiring a larger field of view or more direct access to organs
2. Adhesions (fibrous bands) due to previous surgery or disease process
3. Bleeding
4. Abnormal position of organs.

How often does conversion to open occur?

3–5% of operations.

How are port sites closed?

Rectus sheath/linea alba and Scarpa's fascia need to be closed with absorbable sutures eg PDS. Absorbable skin sutures

What are post-op instructions?

1. Can drink fluids 4 hours post-op, light diet soon after
2. Mobile after 4 hours
3. Home one day post-op (times vary with operation)
4. Routine activity in 5 days
5. Back to work in 10 days.

CHAPTER 9: SUTURES

What is a suture?

A material, synthetic or not, used to appose tissues and facilitate the healing process. It may also be used to ligate blood vessels.

What are the features of the ideal suture?

One that is **non-reactive**, **fully absorbable**, has good **tensile strength-to-thickness properties** (making it strong without undue bulkiness) and has **no memory**. It should maintain its tensile strength until its purpose is served, and should also be **cost-effective**.

What are the different sizes?

Based on the 'O' system: the higher the number of O's, the finer the suture's diameter (eg 4/0 has a smaller diameter than 1/0). The range is: 10/0 to 1/0, then 0, 1, 2, 3, from finest to heaviest.

How are sutures classified?

Mainly as **absorbable** and **non-absorbable**. Also as **synthetic** and **natural**, and **mono-filament** and **braided**.

What sutures do you know of?

(See Table 9.1)

Table 9.1	Synthetic	Natural	
Absorbable	Polydioxanone (*PDS*) Polyglyconate (*Maxon*) *Monocryl*	Catgut	**Mono-filament**
	Polyglactin (*Vicryl*) Polyglycolic acid (*Dexon*)		**Braided**
Non-absorbable	Nylon Prolene Stainless steel	Silk Linen	**Mono-filament**
		Silk	**Braided**

What is catgut made out of?   Sheep's bladder (No cats involved!).

When are the different types of sutures used?

Absorbable: within the body and on the skin.

Non-absorbable: vascular surgery and skin (stainless steel used to close sternum in cardiothoracic surgery).

What is the disadvantage of braided sutures?

Bacteria can theoretically be harboured between strands, thus predisposing to wound infection. However, they have superior strength.

What is the disadvantage of synthetic sutures?

Memory: the suture tends to return to its original straight state, making knot-tying more technically difficult (doesn't **lie** well). Silk (natural) is great knot-tying material as it has almost no memory.

What is the disadvantage of natural sutures?

Cause brisk tissue reaction and have shorter half-life. Catgut also has theoretical risk of causing **prion disease**.

SECTION 2

A. The General Surgical take

CHAPTER 10: THE ACUTE ABDOMEN

APPLIED ANATOMY

What are the landmarks of the foregut, midgut and hindgut, and what is the significance?

Foregut: From the mouth to the ampulla of Vater (mound within 2nd part of duodenum through which CBD drains bile); includes liver, biliary tree and pancreas. Visceral pain from foregut is referred to the **epigastrium.**

Midgut: From ampulla of Vater to distal 1/3 of colon. Visceral pain from midgut is referred to the **periumbilical region.**

Hindgut: From distal 1/3 of colon to anal canal. Visceral pain from the hindgut is referred to the **suprapubic region.**

How is the abdomen sub-divided clinically?

Either into **quadrants:**
- Left and right upper quadrant (LUQ/RUQ)
- Left and right lower quadrant (LLQ/RLQ)

Or into 9 **sub-divisions:**
- Left and right sub-chondrium
- Left and right flank
- Left and right iliac fossa (LIF/RIF)
- Epigastrium
- Peri-umbilical
- Hypogastrium (syn. suprapubis).

What lines are used to divide the abdomen into 9 sub-divisions?

2 vertical lines: each passing through the mid-clavicular points.
2 horizontal lines: the superior one passing through the sub-costal plane (at the tip of the 12th rib), and the inferior one passing through the iliac crests.

What is the main feature of a surgical history?

It is a **pointed** history. Get the facts and get out! Then be able to present the salient points in as few lines as possible (see p. 6 for an example).

What are the important points in the history?

They are as follows:
Pain: usually the main complaint; the following features of pain must be asked about (*know them cold!*);
***mnemonic: SOCRRATES*:**
Site
Onset: sudden, slow
Character: burning, colicky, sharp, dull, cramping
Radiation: vital question!
Relieving factors: analgesia, postural changes, eating, vomiting
Associated symptoms:
The following is a list of important ones:
- *Systemic:* fever +/– rigors, malaise, jaundice, symptoms of anaemia (headaches, lethargy, palpitations)
- *Upper GI:* nausea, vomiting, anorexia, haematemesis (qualify into bright red or coffee-ground vomitus)
- *Lower GI:* constipation, diarrhoea, PR bleed (qualify into bright red, altered/mixed with stool or melaena).

Timing: constant, intermittent (quantify)
Exacerbating factors: posture, movement, coughing, eating
Severity.

Past medical history (PMHx):
anything that may be of importance

to the anaesthetist if an operation is needed (eg HTN, DM).

Past drug history (PDHx): especially anticoagulants such as warfarin or aspirin which may need to be stopped pre-op.

Past surgical history (PSHx): may clue in to a diagnosis (eg SBO 2ry to adhesions from previous laparotomy), or r/o diagnoses (eg acute abdomen is *not* appendicitis in someone who has already had an appendicectomy!).

Family history (FHx): *relevant* history only (eg FAP or IBD).

Social history (SHx): again, *relevant* history only (eg smoking/alcohol/drug habits; living situation: who is at home to care for them on discharge?).

EXAMINATION

How do you begin your examination?

General inspection! In particular, the following will tend to suggest an acute abdomen:
- Patient is unwell-looking (you'll know it when you see it)
- Sweaty (syn. **diaphoretic**)
- Lying still to prevent movement which may aggravate abdominal pain
- Lying with knees up for same reason.

What should be examined in a patient presenting with an acute abdomen and why?

Hands: Sweaty palms (may be cool and clammy if in shock), tachycardia

Face: Sweaty, flushed, mucous membranes (dry if dehydrated, pale if anaemic/bleeding)

Abdomen: Inspect for surgical scars and herniae (ask pt to raise head off bench to exaggerate herniae), and for movements during respiration ($\downarrow$ in peritonitis). **Palpate** for masses (esp. AAA at epigastrium: both **expansile** and **pulsatile**), tenderness (quantify), guarding and rebound tenderness. **Percuss** mainly for rebound tenderness in the acute abdomen. **Auscultate** for bowel sounds ($\uparrow$ in bowel obstruction, $\downarrow$ in peritonitis).

How can rebound be tested?

In several ways:
1. Palpating and then suddenly lifting your hand off the abdomen to see if this causes pain (*not pleasant* for both patients and watchful examiners!)
2. Percussion reproduces pain
3. Asking patient to cough
4. Asking patient to 'blow out your belly and then suck it in'.

INVESTIGATIONS

What investigations should initially be ordered?

Bedside investigations:
1. Urine dipstick (r/o UTI/renal calculi)
2. Pregnancy test in females (r/o gynaecological pathology)
3. Blood sugar level (r/o DKA which can mimic an acute abdomen).

Then what?

Bloods: These will vary according to the presumed cause of the acute abdomen, but *in general* an FBC and U+Es/Cr should always be ordered *first*. Tests like ESR and CRP are generally not of use in the acute situation.

Imaging: Again, these will vary, but *in general* a CXR and AXR should be ordered *first*.

DIFFERENTIAL DIAGNOSES

What is your differential diagnosis mainly based on?

The **history**. Examination and investigations serve only to complement your clinical suspicion.

What differential diagnoses of acute abdomen do you know of?

See Table 10.1

Table 10.1

	Differential diagnosis
Left hypochondrium	Splenic injury
Epigastrium	Peptic ulcer disease Gastritis Pancreatitis/pancreatic abscess Strangulated epigastric hernia Ruptured AAA
Right hypochondrium	Hepatitis Cholecystitis Empyema of the gallbladder
Left and right flanks	Pyelonephritis/pyonephrosis Renal calculi Distended ascending/descending colon (in LBO)
Periumbilicus	Distended small bowel (in SBO) Strangulated (peri)umbilical hernia
Left iliac fossa	Diverticulitis/diverticular abscess Distended descending colon (in LBO) Mittelschmirtz Torsion of ovarian cyst Salpingo-oophoritis
Suprapubis	Diverticulitis/diverticular abscess Distended bladder Pelvic inflammatory disease (PID) Torsion of uterine fibroid

Table 10.1 (continued)

	Differential diagnosis
Right iliac fossa	Appendicitis
	Terminal ileitis (in Crohn's disease)
	Distended caecum (in LBO)
	Mittelschmirtz
	Torsion of ovarian cyst
	Salpingo-oophoritis

What medical causes of acute abdominal pain must you be aware of?

Diabetic ketoacidosis and sickle cell crisis

How can the causes of RIF pain be remembered?

mnemonic: **APPENDICITIS**
Appendicitis/ **A**bscess
PID/**P**eriod
Pancreatitis
Ectopic pregnancy/**E**ndometriosis
Neoplasia
Diverticulitis
Intussusception
Cyst (ovarian)
IBD eg Crohn's disease
Torsion (ovary)
Irritable bowel syndrome
Stones.

TREATMENT

How would you manage an acute abdomen?

Depends on the clinical diagnosis, but in *all* patients, *resuscitate first!*
1. Admit
2. **Rule of tubes!**
   a. Oxygen mask
   b. IV access with fluids (and take bloods simultaneously)
   c. Urinary catheter
   d. NG tube (as necessary).
Then *and only then* do you think about further treatment. The priority is to stabilise the patient.

What is peritonitis? Inflammation of the peritoneum.

What types do you know of? Primary and secondary.
Primary: usually due to seeding haematogenous bacterial spread (eg spontaneous bacterial peritonitis [infection of ascitic fluid] and tuberculous peritonitis).
Secondary: usually due to a perforated viscus (eg perforated peptic ulcer or burst appendix). Bile leakage from a ruptured gallbladder or from the biliary tree post exploration may cause a **chemical peritonitis** which is initially sterile, but may become super-infected.

What are the symptoms of peritonitis? Fever, malaise, nausea, vomiting, generalised severe abdominal pain, and unwillingness to move as movement aggravates pain.

What are the clinical findings? *General:* ill-looking patient, lying still and sweating; febrile; may be actively vomiting.
Hands: sweaty; tachycardia
Abdomen: **inspection:** no movements with respiration; **palpation:** generalised tenderness (may be localised if pathology is confined to one area, as in burst appendix) and **board-like rigidity**; rebound and guarding present; **percussion:** rebound tenderness; **auscultation:** absent bowel sounds.
Rectal: nil specific; rectum may be hot.

What is the management? Actively resuscitate the patient (see above) and treat the underlying cause.

What are the spot diagnoses in the following clinical scenarios?

Peri-umbilical to RIF pain associated with fever and anorexia in a 15 y.o. boy?	Acute appendicitis.
LIF pain with fever and a raised WBC in a 65 y.o. woman with altered bowel habit?	Acute diverticulitis.
RUQ pain radiating to epigastrium and right scapular tip associated with fever in a 45 y.o. woman?	Acute cholecystitis.
Shock in a 85 y.o. man with a pulsatile abdominal mass?	Ruptured abdominal aortic aneurysm.
Pain aggravated by eating, and out proportion to palpation in a 70 y.o. smoker?	Mesenteric ischaemia (syn. **abdominal angina**).
RIF pain associated with vaginal bleeding in a 20 y.o. girl?	Ruptured ectopic pregnancy.

CHAPTER 11: THE TRAUMA CALL

What are the principles of ATLS?

Advanced **T**rauma **L**ife **S**upport principles advocate a thorough and reliable system of examination and initial resuscitation in order to identify and immediately treat potentially fatal injuries in trauma, followed by a more thorough and detailed assessment of the whole body leading eventually to complete and definitive care. These two processes are divided into a **primary** and **secondary** survey.

What is the primary survey?

It is the initial assessment of the trauma patient, designed to identify and treat life-threatening injuries immediately so that initial resuscitation is maximally effective. Remember assess **A, B, C, D and E:**
- **A**irway and cervical spine immobilisation
- **B**reathing (respiratory system)
- **C**irculation and haemorrhage control (cardiovascular system)
- **D**isability
- **E**xposure.

What life-threatening factors *must* be identified and treated in the primary survey?

mnemonic: **ATOMIC**
Airway compromise resulting in inadequate ventilation
Tension pneumothorax
Open pneumothorax/sucking chest wound
Massive haemothorax
Incipient flail chest
Cardiac tamponade.

What are the aims of the secondary survey?

A thorough head to toe assessment after initial resuscitation to identify all injuries caused by trauma and outline a plan for full treatment and definitive care.

What X-rays are included in a standard trauma series?

The following films:
1. Lateral C-spine
2. CXR
3. Pelvic XR.

THE PRIMARY SURVEY

AIRWAY AND C-SPINE CONTROL

Who is at risk of C-spine injury and subsequent neurological damage?

All patients involved in trauma must be assumed to have an unstable C-spine # until excluded clinically and radiologically.

How is the C-spine initially managed?

In the following ways:
1. **C-spine hard collar**: reduces voluntary movement by around 30%.
2. **Bilateral sandbags/struts** taped across bed to secure hard collar in fixed position. Suboptimal immobilisation in a hard collar is only used in a restless agitated patient, as this is preferred to splinting the C-spine of a thrashing torso/lower body.

How is the C-spine definitively managed?

With radiological assessment which includes the following three views:
1. Lateral C-spine: picks up 80% of C-spine injuries. Must include all 7 cervical vertebrae *and* the C7–T1 junction to be an **adequate film**
2. AP view – picks up 95% of bony injuries when combined with the lateral view
3. Open mouth/odontoid peg view – picks up 99% of injuries when used with above views. Further management is based on findings.

What types of injuries compromise the airway?

Two main groups:

1. **Facial/neck trauma:** stab wounds to the neck, facial trauma post-assault or unrestrained passengers in head-on collisions, causing oropharyngeal loose bodies/haematoma/ bruising.

2. **Head injury with low GCS and impaired laryngeal/pharyngeal reflexes:** GCS < 8 with impaired cough or gag reflex implies inability to self protect the airway against aspiration of vomit/blood. The airway must therefore be cleared and secured.

How is the airway evaluated?

Ask a simple question. A lucid response in a normal voice implies an intact airway with no laryngeal compromise. If no response:

Look: for any misting of the oxygen mask, facial trauma, blood or foreign bodies in the oropharynx and signs of any ventilatory obstruction, such as tracheal tug, see saw breathing (abdominal retraction on inspiration with no chest movement) or complete apnoea/cyanosis.

Listen: for signs of air movement, cough reflex and evidence of upper airway obstruction such as:

- Stridor (hoarse inspiratory sound caused by extrathoracic large airway obstruction)
- Gurgling
- Wheeze (expiratory sound caused by intrathoracic small airway obstruction – implies pathology within chest rather than at airway level).

Feel: for breath on your cheek; assess chest expansion/symmetry at

How is tension pneumot[horax] treated?

What are the anatomica[l] landmarks for thoracocentesis?

What are the anatomica[l] landmarks for chest dra[in] insertion?

How is open pneumotho[rax] treated?

What further investigations should be obtained?	**Blood investigations:**
	1. GXM: for transfusion as necessary
	2. ABG: provides invaluable information regarding oxygenation and lung function as well as an **immediate Hb estimation**. Can also provide **carboxyhaemoglobin** estimation in cases of smoke inhalation.
	Imaging:
	1. CXR: still the most important, mandatory investigation in all trauma patients:
	Pneumothorax: loss of outer lung markings (1 cm rim of lucency approx. = to 10% loss of lung volume).
	Haemothorax: blunting of costophrenic angle on erect chest implies 300–400 ml blood in the pleural space. Also in diagnosis of contusion, parenchymal injury and other pathology.
	2. CT scan: used as necessary to provide specific information only in a patient stable for transfer and after the secondary survey.
How are these conditic detected clinically?	

CIRCULATION

What is shock?	Shock is the clinically used term for a **compromise in circulation** leading to **inadequate tissue perfusion**. Metabolic demands of the body are not met leading to abnormal physiology.
What types of shock are there?	There are five types:
	1. **Hypovolaemic:** low intravascular volume eg in haemorrhage
	2. **Cardiogenic:** failure of the heart as a pumping mechanism due to

1ry damage and/or 2ry cardiac tamponade
3. **Septic:** maldistribution of fluid due to the action of chemical messengers during the inflammatory process of infection
4. **Neurogenic:** maldistribution of fluid due to loss of muscle tone/nerve signals; eg in transection of the spinal cord
5. **Anaphylactic:** maldistribution of fluid due to allergic stimulus and cytokine release.

What do they all have in common?

Intravascular fluid volume is no longer adequate to transport oxygen to the tissues for cellular uptake and aerobic metabolism.

In a shocked patient, which type is assumed until proven otherwise?

Hypovolaemic 2ry to haemorrhage.

What types of haemorrhage do you know?

There are two types:
1. **Obvious haemorrhage:**
   • Compound fractures
   • Digital/limb amputation
   • Arterial puncture wounds.
2. **'Hidden' haemorrhage:**
   • Long bone fractures (closed)
   • Thoracic trauma (collects in thoracic cavity)
   • Abdominal trauma (intra/extra-peritoneal)
   • Pelvic fractures (closed).

Which wounds must be treated with a high index of suspicion?

Penetrating wounds to the neck and mediastinum (risk of large vessel puncture or cardiac puncture leading to tamponade or cardiogenic shock).

How is shock clinically assessed?

Look:
• Peripheral/central cyanosis (↓perfusion)

- Patient cold and clammy (**'shut down'** due to peripheral vasoconstriction as a sympathetic response to haemorrhage)
- Distended jugular veins (cardiogenic shock)
- Visible trauma with/without haemorrhage
- Respiratory rate (normally 14–20 in adult)
- Evidence of confusion, aggression, drowsiness or coma (cerebral hypoxia)
- Jugular venous pulse (JVP) wave if present (this is a tricky sign in any situation and so its use in the rapid assessment of a trauma patient is minimal).

Listen:
- Muffled heart sounds over the appropriate areas

Feel:
- Pulse: note **rate** (normal 60–100), **rhythm** (regular/ irregular) and **volume** (bounding, thready, absent). If radial pulse absent, try carotid and femoral arteries. No pulse indicates **cardiac arrest** and BLS should be commenced.
- Capillary refill time (CRT): press on sternum for 5 seconds. The area should blanch and return to normal colour in less than 2 seconds. Longer implies shock.

What *must* also be performed?

The following bedside investigations:
- Blood pressure
- Oxygen saturations
- Cardiac monitoring and rhythm trace

• Urine output (usually as part of the secondary survey post catheterisation).

How can this information be used to assess blood loss in a patient in haemorrhagic shock?

See Table 11.1. It is based on the average 70 kg man with a 5 litre intravascular volume.

Table 11.1

	Class 1	Class 2	Class 3	Class 4
BP Systolic Diastolic	Unchanged Unchanged	Normal Raised	Reduced Reduced	Very low Very low/ unrecordable
Pulse bpm Volume	High normal Normal	100–120 Normal	>120 Thready	>120 Very thready
CRT	Normal	Slow (>2 s)	Slow (>2 s)	Undetectable
Respiratory rate	Normal	Tachypnoea	>20/min	>20/min
Urine output	>30 ml/h	20–30 ml/h	10–20 ml/h	0–10 ml/h
Extremities	Normal colour	Pale	Pale	Pale, clammy
Complexion	Normal	Pale	Pale	Ashen
Mental state	Alert	Anxious	Aggressive/ drowsy	Drowsy/ confused
Blood loss (*like game of tennis*) % Volume	*Love–fifteen* <15% 750 ml	*Fifteen–thirty* 15–30% 800–1500 ml	*Thirty–forty* 30–40% 1500–2000 ml	*Game over!* >40% >2000 ml

How is shock managed?

As hypovolaemic shock until proven otherwise: with rapid intravascular volume repletion (fluids).

So how would you treat this?

In the following steps:
1. Intravenous access via two wide bore cannulae (14 G ideally) in the antecubital fossa

2. *Failing this*: cannulation of any forearm veins with the widest bore possible
3. *Failing this*: a surgical 'cut down' (direct exposure of an accessible vein via dissection); saphenous vein most commonly used
4. *In kids, if 1 & 2* fail: intraosseus access can be attempted at the tibial tuberosity (*not* adults!)

NB Immediate central venous access with a large bore cannula or via the Seldinger technique may be used first in experienced hands. Otherwise, it is used when peripheral access is impossible.

Initial replacement should then be commenced with a 10–20 ml/kg bolus of warmed fluid via a pressure bag.

What is your 1st choice of fluid?

Hartmann's solution.

What is the Seldinger technique?

A needle is inserted into a central vein (jugular or subclavian), and a guidewire is threaded through it. Needle is removed, and a cannula is threaded over the wire into the vein and secured.

What should be done after cannulation but *before* starting fluids?

Collect 20 ml blood for:
1. G&S (or GXM depending on clinical scenario)
2. FBC: baseline
3. U&Es: baseline
4. Glucose estimation (via BM machine preferentially or lab glucose)
5. Serum save (for future tests as needed, forensic or otherwise).

What else must also be done?

The following adjunctive measures:

1. Adequate oxygenation (hence why B comes before C in the ABCDEs!). No benefit in restoring circulation if hypoxia continues, due to inadequate ventilation/oxygenation of blood at lungs): give as much O_2 therapy as possible, via intubation if necessary.
2. Control of external haemorrhage:
   - Direct pressure onto bleeding area
   - Elevation of injured limb
   - Head-down tilt to maximise cerebral perfusion.

What types of fluids are used in shock?

The following are available:

1. Hartmann's solution (syn. **Ringer's lactate**)
2. Other crystalloids (eg normal saline)
3. Colloids (gelatin solutions): high osmotic load thought to give greater intravascular volume expansion
4. Blood products: provide oxygen transport, unlike any of above fluids.

When is blood indicated?

In ongoing fluid loss and with class 3–4 shock (30–40% blood loss).

What type of blood should be used?

Depends on the clinical scenario and condition of the patient on arrival:
Needed immediately: O–ve (universal donor)
- Packed rhesus negative (Rh–ve) type O red cells with no surface AB antigen and no anti A or anti B plasma
- Not cross-matched, therefore mild/moderate transfusion

reactions unrelated to ABO rhesus system may occur

Needed quickly (5–10 min): Type specific

- ABO typed to match recipient's blood type
- Not fully cross-matched for other antigens
- Requires serum sample of pt's blood to the lab

Needed within 30–60 min: Fully cross-matched

- ABO and antibody screened to ensure maximum compatibility with recipient
- Requires serum sample of pt's blood to the lab.

Once initial shock treatment has begun, what next?

Directed treatment of the actual cause of shock.

What life threatening circulatory condition must be identified and treated during the 1ry survey?

Cardiac tamponade: accumulation of blood within the fibrous pericardial sac (usually 2ry to myocardial trauma). This exerts external pressure on the heart and interferes with diastolic filling and subsequent ventricular ejection.

How is cardiac tamponade recognized?

Beck's Triad:
1. Hypotension
2. Muffled heart sounds
3. Raised JVP

Also, **Kussmaul's sign**: raised JVP on inspiration due to impeded venous return.

What is cardiac tamponade a diagnosis of?

Exclusion. Usually diagnosed when inserting bilateral chest drains for a haemothorax results in no clinical improvement.

What is the management of cardiac tamponade?

ABCs (*always say this first!*), followed by 1 of 2 options:
1. Emergency pericardiocentesis (aspiration of blood from pericardial sac)
2. Emergency room thoracotomy (open evacuation of pericardial sac +/− 1ry repair of wound).

When should a ER thoracotomy be done?

In the following circumstances:
1. Penetrating trauma to the chest (especially pericardiac) with established vital signs initially, followed by marked clinical deterioration.
2. Uncontrollable life-threatening intra-hilar haemorrhage, requiring cross clamping as an emergency measure prior to theatre.

What are the contraindications?

Numerous, but include:
- Blunt trauma
- >10 min CPR
- All patients with no established vital signs at the scene.

DISABILITY

How would you immediately assess neurological status?

The **AVPU** system in the immediate, followed by the definitive Glasgow Coma Scale (**GCS**):
AVPU:
A: spontaneously **A**lert (equivalent to GCS 14–15)
V: responsive to **V**oice (equivalent to GCS 9–10)
P: responsive to **P**ain (equivalent to GCS 7–8)
U: **U**nresponsive (equivalent to GCS of 3).

GCS: comprises three elements and is scored by best possible response to give a total out of 15:

Best eye response
- No response [1]
- Eye opening to painful stimuli [2]
- Eye opening to verbal stimuli [3]
- Spontaneous eye opening [4]

Best verbal response
- No verbal response [1]
- Incomprehensible (noises) [2]
- Inappropriate (words only) [3]
- Confused (talking in sentences) [4]
- Orientated and lucid response [5]

Best motor response
- No response [1]
- Decerebrate [2]
- Decorticate [3]
- Withdrawal to pain [4]
- Localising to pain [5]
- Following commands [6]

What is the highest GCS score?	15: pt. fully alert, awake and aware.
What is the lowest GCS score?	3 (*not zero!*): pt. comatose/unresponsive.
At what GCS score should a patient be intubated?	8
How often should the GCS be repeated in trauma?	Every 15 minutes. Document every time!

EXPOSURE

How much of the patient should be exposed?	**All!** The patient should be fully exposed from head to toe to note any injuries at any points on the body (use shears if necessary).
Why?	Visual clues may exist after full exposure eg seatbelt marks indicating possible sternal trauma.

What *must* be done on exposure?	A log-roll (pt. rolled onto side whilst maintaining spinal immobility; requires up to 5 people).
What is assessed on log-roll?	Back, buttocks, thighs and posterior legs and spine (deformities, focal tenderness, ecchymoses). A DRE *must* be done.
What information is gained on DRE?	1. Anal tone ($\downarrow$ in cord trauma) 2. Blood (anorectal/pelvic trauma) 3. Prostate (high-riding prostate suggests urethral rupture) 4. Bony spicules (pelvic fracture).
What must be avoided in the exposed patient?	Hypothermia. Insulation is a *must* following log-roll.
How is core body temperature most accurately assessed?	Rectally.

How can core temperature be raised in hypothermia?	1. Bair huggers™ and covering (mild hypothermia)
	2. Warmed fluid instituted into bodily orifices:
	  • IV fluids
	  • Orogastric
	  • Intravesical
	  • Intraperitoneal
	  • Rectal.

SECONDARY SURVEY

What are the essential objectives of the secondary survey?	Having addressed and treated any immediate life-threatening injuries, the secondary survey refers to a definitive history, thorough examination and formation of a management plan: • Examination from head to toe, front and back • 'Fingers and tubes in every orifice' • Incident and collateral history

- Complete medical history
- Assimilation of all directed investigations
- Formulation of a definitive management plan.

What investigations should be done in the secondary survey?

Any relevant ones. At the very least a trauma series should be obtained, together with basic blood tests and an ECG.

What history should you take?

1. Paramedic handover
2. Collateral witness history
3. Patient's history
4. **AMPLE** medical history
   Allergies
   Medications
   Past medical history
   Last meal
   Events leading to situation.

What happens if a change or deterioration in a patient's clinical condition occurs?

Return to assessment of ABCDE immediately and evaluate/treat as necessary until the patient's stability allows them to proceed to the secondary survey.

HEAD AND CNS

What are the key abnormalities on scalp/ occiput examination?

Remember: the more visible injury, the more invisible (intracranial) injury may be present. Any lacerations should be cleaned, assessed and closed if possible. Key points:
History
- Mechanism of injury (penetrating, missile, blunt trauma)
- Tetanus immunisation status
- Time elapsed since injury.
Clean and explore
- Foreign bodies
- Dirt in wound

- Exploration to assess length and depth
- Boggy swelling suggesting underlying #.

Is a skull X-ray indicated?
- High velocity injury
- Assault with a weapon
- Marked bruising or extensive laceration
- Any focal neurological deficit or drop in GCS.

Is it an open #?
- Is there a bony # underneath the wound, implying direct contact between body surface and cranial vault?
- Requires neurosurgical consultation
- Take advice before closing
- May need IV antibiotics and continued observation.

Can it be closed in the resus room?
- If deterioration demands transfer, control with pressure dressings is preferred to delay
- Scalp avulsions may require plastic surgery opinion
- Close with non-adsorbable sutures if appropriate, or staples for speed.

What is meant by 1ry and 2ry brain injury?

Primary brain injury: initial brain injury sustained at time of incident due to direct trauma/mechanical insult

Secondary brain injury: continuing damage to cerebral tissue caused by an altered chemical environment and/or impaired physiology; causes:
- Hypoxaemia
- Hypercarbia
- Hypotension.

What intracranial lesions must be considered in a closed head injury (no laceration apparent)?

Skull #: suggested by high impact injury with boggy swelling at site

Basal skull #: suggested by the following signs:

- Panda eyes
- Haemotympanum (blood behind the eardrum)
- CSF rhinorrhoea
- Battle's sign (mastoid bruising).

Extra-dural haematoma:

- Haematoma collecting between skull vault and dural layer of meninges
- Causes raised ICP and deteriorating neurological function
- Often caused by damage to the middle meningeal artery running through the temporal skull
- Often needs surgical evacuation via burr hole or craniotomy/bone flap.

Subdural haematoma: haematoma under the dura but above the arachnoid layer, often caused by shearing of cortical draining veins.

Sub-arachnoid haemorrhage/ intracerebral bleed: bleeding into the sub-arachnoid space/brain substance.

Coup and contre-coup: as the brain is mobile in a fluid-filled cavity, rapid deceleration can cause injury/contusion at the point of impact, with rebound injury at the opposite side.

Diffuse axonal injury: may cause varying degrees of amnesia.

What are the indications for a skull X-ray?

Considered when a CT head will not be performed, but concerns regarding skull fractures or intracranial trauma exist:

- High velocity injury
- Focal neurological signs
- Loss of consciousness or any alteration in conscious level post injury
- Marked superficial trauma.

What are the indications for a CT scan of the head?

Immediate CT scanning is suggested in the following situations:
- Vomiting >2 episodes post head injury
- Focal neurological signs
- GCS <13 at any time since injury
- GCS 13/14 two hours post-injury
- Post traumatic seizure
- Any signs of a basal skull #/open skull #
- Loss of consciousness or amnesia in patients >65 or with any coagulopathy.

CT scanning is also recommended within 8 hours for those patients with none of the above, but with a history of retrograde amnesia >30 min or loss of consciousness, with a dangerous mechanism of injury (RTA or fall >5 m).

What is the management of severe head injury?

In severe head injury either clinically or as picked up by CT scan, do the following:
- Intubation and ventilation
- Maintenance of normocarbia
- Prophylactic antibiotics for open/basal skull #
- IV mannitol to decrease ICP/steroids usually given on the advice of neurosurgical consult
- Urgent neurosurgical opinion.

How is a patient with potential spinal injury immobilised?

1. Hard collar: prevents flexion/ extension
2. Sandbags with in line

stabilisation: prevents lateral flexion/rotation

3. Spinal board: used for extraction from hostile environment.

How should a stabilised C-spine be approached?

Above all do no harm. Patients should remain in C-spine immobilisation until fully investigated and assessed:

History: including mechanism of injury, symptoms, previous injuries or operations on spine

Clinical exam:

- Full PNS exam should be performed to evaluate potential uni/bilateral weakness, paraesthesiae, hyperreflexia, hypertonia, and other signs suggestive of spinal cord injury
- With the C-spine manually immobilised by an assistant, the hard collar is removed and the spine palpated for any bony abnormalities (steps or swelling), subjective pain, and tenderness. Spinal movements should not be evaluated here. Full spinal precautions should be replaced after the exam.

What C-spine films would you order?

AP, lateral, and odontoid peg films.

What *must* you be able to see on the lateral film?

Film *must* include C7/T1 junction. If this cannot be adequately obtained due to patient's condition, two options exist:

- Manual traction on the patient's arms inferiorly and repeat
- Swimmer's view/trauma oblique – shoot through with shoulder abducted to 140°.

| **What if this *still* doesn't work?** | CT scan of the C-spine (often performed with the cranial scan). |

ABDOMEN

| **When is abdominal trauma assessed?** | After ABCDEs have been stabilised! |

How should abdominal examination be approached in the secondary survey?

Above all, be systematic.
The essentials are detailed below.

Look:
- Full exposure of abdomen/flanks/back and perineum
- Evidence of blunt/penetrating injury
- 'Fullness' implying distension
- Penetrating objects should *not* be removed blindly in A&E.

Listen:
- Bowel sounds
- Renal or aortic bruits (?traumatic aneurysm/rupture).

Feel:
- For tenderness/rebound/guarding/masses in all quadrants
- Rectal examination:
    1. For signs of possible urethral injury (see below)
    2. For signs of rectal injury (blood in rectum, loss of wall integrity).
- Vaginal examination in females:
    1. Confirms integrity of vaginal wall
    2. Detects obvious pelvic fractures.
- Pass nasogastric tube:
    1. Decompression of stomach and aspiration of gastric contents to limit risk of aspiration
    2. May give valuable clue to gastric injury if blood is aspirated.

- Pass urethral catheter unless signs suggesting urethral injury exist:
  1. High riding prostate
  2. Blood at the urethral meatus
  3. Bruising of the perineum and/or scrotum.

What basic investigations are mandatory for abdominal trauma?

The principle of abdominal investigation revolves around resuscitation of ABC, and the attempt to decide whether the patient needs a laparotomy or not.

Blood investigations:
1. GXM
2. Baseline FBC/U&Es/LFT/amylase
3. ABG to determine any metabolic acidosis
4. Pregnancy testing in all females of a reproductive age.

Radiography:
1. Erect CXR: to evaluate free intra-peritoneal air
2. Pelvic XR
3. AXR if possibility of embedded foreign bodies exists

In severe intra-abdominal injury, urgent laparotomy is considered without formal investigation.

What are the indications for urgent laparotomy?

1. Evisceration (bowel protrusion through abdominal wall)
2. All gunshot wounds
3. Unexplained shock
4. Rigid and silent abdomen
5. Free air under the diaphragm on erect CXR.

What other investigations can be considered to assess the extent of abdominal trauma?

If the patient has no immediate indication for a laparotomy, but displays obvious evidence of abdominal trauma, the following can be done to help with the decision to operate or not:

1. **Ultrasonography**
   - Portable to the patient (no need for transfer)
   - Can identify free fluid in the abdomen primarily
   - Can be operated by surgical/casualty staff, with appropriate training.

2. **CT scanning**
   - Requires stability of the patient and transfer
   - Particularly useful in identifying organ damage and cause of free fluid
   - Needs formal radiological interpretation.

3. **Diagnostic peritoneal lavage (DPL)**
   - Offers a reliable indicator of intestinal perforation/intra-abdominal haemorrhage without formal laparotomy or transfer
   - Useful in the following situations:
   1. Unreliable clinical exam
   2. Unexplained hypotension/hypovolaemia
   3. If the patient is undergoing lengthy extra-abdominal procedures.

How is DPL performed?

A catheter insertion into an incision in the midline of the lower abdominal wall (bladder must be emptied first) and aspiration is performed, noting any blood or faeculent products. 10 ml/kg of warmed saline is irrigated through the catheter and mixed gently (rock abdomen from side to side). The fluid is aspirated after 10 min and sent for laboratory evaluation of effluent.

What is a positive DPL result?

The following:
- >5 ml frank blood on initial aspiration
- Obvious intestinal matter
- >100,000 red blood cells/mm^3 in lavage fluid
- >500 white blood cells/mm^3 in lavage fluid.

What are the contra-indications for DPL?

Absolute: definite need for a laparotomy
Relative:
- Gross obesity
- Advanced pregnancy
- Coagulopathy
- Previous surgery
- Known ascites.

What causes of intra-abdominal bleeding do you know?

The most important ones are listed here:
Hepatic injury:
- Laceration, haematoma or hepatic vascular injury
- Graded according to severity/lobar involvement
- Surgery vs. conservative treatment depends on haemodynamic status and grade of injury
- Surgery consists of packing and tamponade effect rather than direct suturing of parenchyma.

Splenic trauma:
- Laceration, haematoma or splenic vascular injury
- Graded according to severity/site
- Surgery vs. conservative treatment depends on haemodynamic status and grade of injury
- More effort being made to attempt to save the spleen where possible, to prevent later complications such as overwhelming sepsis after splenectomy

- Conservative treatment requires haemodynamic stability after resuscitation (>2 units transfusion needed in adults implies need for splenectomy) and facilities for intensive observation +/– urgent surgery if needed
- Surgery: splenic/vascular repair or total splenectomy
- Pneumococcal and Hib vaccination, with prophylactic penicillin (at least 2 years) should follow splenectomy.

Small bowel injury:
- May follow penetrating injury or rupture/burst with blunt trauma
- Detected well by DPL but often difficult to identify with imaging
- Surgery: defect repair, or resection with primary anastomosis if the injured section appears non-viable at surgery
- Mesenteric tears can result in impaired blood supply and resultant bowel ischaemia.

Colorectal injury:
- As with small bowel injury
- Primary anastomosis often avoided with gross faecal leak due to breakdown and subsequent intra-abdominal sepsis
- Stoma often created while patient recovers from other traumatic injuries.

Pancreatic injury:
- Uncommon in isolation due to retroperitoneal positioning
- Suggested by an elevated serum amylase
- Often discovered at laparotomy
- Pancreatography often needed to delineate the extent of duct injury.

What is the relevant history? Ask about the following:

Penetrating injury:

1. Usually of the upper urinary tract
2. Gunshot/stab wounds.

Blunt injury:

1. Can be upper or lower urinary tract
2. RTA/deceleration injuries usually cause renal injury compression between the ribs and spine
3. Lower urinary tract injury includes intra/extraperitoneal bladder rupture and bulbar urethral injury following direct trauma to perineum.

What are the exam findings? Keep the following in mind:

Visual inspection:

1. Penetrating wounds
2. Surrounding bony injuries (ribs/pelvis)
3. Loin swelling/bruising
4. Scrotal degloving/laceration
5. 'Butterfly haematoma': bruising confined to **Colles fascia**, from collection of extravasated blood and urine in the perineum.

Palpation:

1. Loin tenderness
2. Loss of loin contour
3. PR exam (high riding prostate = uretheral rupture)
4. Scrotal haematoma.

What different parts of the urethra must be considered? In the male, the urethra is divided into 4 areas dependent on its surrounding structures:

1. Prostatic urethra
2. Membranous urethra
3. Bulbar urethra
4. Penile urethra.

The female urethra is 4 cm long and acts as an external sphincter for the bladder. It is usually spared from injury, unless subjected to direct trauma.

What *must* accompany examination in suspected urinary tract trauma?

Urinalysis: ideally via micturition, but via catheter if necessary, *assuming there are no signs of urethral injury contra-indicating catheterisation*, looking for any macro- or microscopic haematuria implying urinary tract injury.

What signs suggest urethral injury?

1. High riding, mobile prostate on DRE
2. Blood at the urethral meatus
3. Inability to void
4. Perineal bruising.

When would you consider a urethral catheter in trauma?

Only if there are no signs of urethral injury and DRE is normal. Otherwise, a **suprapubic catheter** should be considered.

How is suspected *upper* urinary tract trauma investigated?

With one or more of the following methods:

1. **Intravenous urography:** readily available and transportable to patient; do preliminary control film (KUB) first:
   - Abnormalities seen in 15% of cases of blunt renal trauma
   - Include loss of psoas shadow or renal outline (indicates bleeding), # ribs

   IV contrast followed by series of films at later intervals monitoring excretion:
   - 85% show no abnormalities
   - May see extravasation of dye, pelvicaliceal disruption or absence of caliceal system

- Can be compared to contralateral non-injured side.
2. **Renal ultrasonography:** readily available and transportable to the patient; can be used to identify:
   - Parenchymal disruption
   - Haematomas (subcapsular/intra-renal)
   - Peri-renal collections.
3. **CT scanning:** gives similar information to above methods when used together; can provide other information in blunt abdominal trauma, but requires patient transfer and therefore stabilisation.
4. **Selective renal arteriography:** indicated in macroscopic haematuria persisting >1 week.

What percentage of blunt renal tract injuries are life-threatening?

Less than 5%.

How is confirmed upper urinary tract trauma managed then?

ABCs and treatment of serious pathology as a priority. Once stabilised and investigated, renal pathology can be treated.

What are the treatment options?

Can be surgical or non-surgical:
Surgical exploration: Mandatory in the following:
1. Penetrating stab/gunshot wounds with high grade renal trauma
2. Patients with critical or unstable major closed renal injuries.
May be indicated for late complications for any renal injury, including AV fistula, hydronephrosis or chronic pyelonephritis.

Conservative treatment: initially appropriate for 95% closed renal trauma. Comprises:

1. Bed rest
2. Analgesia
3. Prophylactic antibiotics
4. Serial reassessment.

How is suspected *lower* urinary tract trauma investigated?

With one or more of the following methods:

1. **Plain pelvic X-ray:** looking for any evidence of pelvic fractures with associated bladder puncture by bony fragments
2. **Ascending urethrography:** initial investigation if any suspicion of urethral injury; dye injected up a catheter inserted into the *distal* part of the urethra only. Oblique X-rays taken during study will note extravasation of contrast; if positive, urethral catheterisation is contra-indicated
3. **Catheterisation and cystography:** aims to identify any peritoneal leak of contrast; *performed only if signs of urethral injury excluded*
4. **Intravenous urography:** can also detect bladder perforation/displacement
5. **CT scanning.**

How is confirmed lower urinary tract trauma managed?

Early urological referral.
Bladder rupture: may be intra- or extraperitoneal:

- **Intraperitoneal rupture:** laparotomy and repair; subsequent drainage with both suprapubic and urethral catheter for 7 days; broad spectrum antibiotics
- **Extraperitoneal rupture:** conservatively treated with catheter drainage; cystography to confirm healing prior to catheter removal.

Urethral injury: *do not pass a urethral catheter!* Passing one may:

1. Introduce superinfection
2. May prevent haematoma drainage
3. May pass through tear and create false passage
4. May produce fistula on withdrawal
5. May convert partial to full tear on balloon inflation.

In a **conscious** patient passing urine:

1. Analgesia
2. Antibiotic prophylaxis
3. Urology follow-up as outpatient.

In a **conscious** patient in **retention** or an **unconscious** patient:

1. Suprapubic catheterisation indicated
2. Prophylactic antibiotics
3. Urology follow-up +/− further urethral radiology studies.

CHAPTER 12: APPENDICITIS

APPLIED ANATOMY

Figure 12.1 The appendix

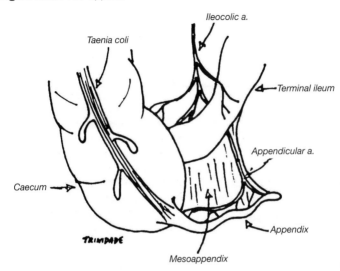

Where is the appendix?	Attached to the end of the caecum.
What is its usual position?	The posteromedial position.
What is its blood supply?	The appendiceal artery, a branch of the ileocolic artery.
Where does it run?	The free edge of the mesoappendix (mesentery of the appendix).
What is appendicitis?	Acute inflammation of the appendix usually **caused by luminal obstruction.**
What are the causes?	Most common cause is a **faecolith** obstructing the lumen; causes can be divided into: **Luminal:** faecolith, worms, seeds **Mural:** lymphoid hyperplasia, Crohn's disease CA, vascular disease of appendiceal a., carcinoid

Extraluminal: caecal tumour, peritonitis.

APPENDICITIS

What is the incidence in the UK?	Approximately 80,000/year.
How does it present?	Periumbilical to RIF pain, nausea and vomiting, fever, **anorexia.**
What is the significance of periumbilical to RIF pain?	Appendix is a **midgut** structure, so pain is 1st **referred** to periumbilical region (**visceral pain**). With continued inflammation, ischaemia occurs, mural nerve endings die and referred pain stops. **Localised** RIF pain now occurs due to irritation of overlying peritoneum by inflamed appendix (**somatic pain**).
How is it diagnosed?	History and examination; acute appendicitis is a **clinical diagnosis.**
What is important when taking history from a female?	A gynaecological history: LNMP, menstrual cycle, sexual history, use of OCP, vaginal bleeding (ectopic pregnancy) or discharge (PID).
What are the relevant clinical findings?	*General:* Febrile, flushed appearance, lying still *Hands:* Clammy, tachycardic *Face:* Fetor oris (distinctive odour to the breath), **coated tongue** *Abdomen:* Rebound/guarding in RIF, especially at McBurney's point (see p. 23).
What special signs do you know of?	Rovsing's sign, obturator sign and psoas sign (see pp. 23, 24).
What are the differential diagnoses?	*Pain from nearby structures:* [Bowel] Meckel's diverticulum (see below), Crohn's disease (terminal ileitis), caecal tumour, intussusception **(ileocaecal);** [Gynae] **ruptured**

ectopic pregnancy, mittleschmerz (ovulation pain), salpingitis, PID, torsion of ovarian cyst; [Urological] ureteric stone, **UTI;** [Abdominal wall] psoas abscess, herpes zoster.
Other differentials: perforated peptic ulcer pancreatitis, cholecystitis, mesenteric adenitis, pyelonephritis.

What investigations should be performed?	**Urine dipstick:** to rule out UTI (leucocytes) and calculi (blood) **Urine pregnancy test [β-HCG]:** to rule out ectopic pregnancy **FBC:** mild leucocytosis (90%), often with a neutrophilia (75%) **USS:** in women where diagnosis is unsure.

What is the management?

1. Admit to ward
2. IV fluids
3. IV analgesia (opiates)
4. IV antibiotics (3rd generation cephalosporin)
5. NBM
6. Consent for an appendicectomy.

How long would you give IV antibiotics for?

If appendix is non-perforated, give 1 dose intra-op and 2 doses post-op; if perforated, continue for 5–7 days post-op.

How is an appendicectomy performed?

Either open or laparoscopically.

In open appendicectomy, what layers do you go through?

1. Skin
2. Subcutaneous fat
3. Camper's fascia
4. Scarpa's fascia
5. External oblique
6. Internal oblique
7. Transversus abdominis
8. Transversalis fascia
9. Peritoneum.

How do you find the base of the appendix at operation?

Follow the taeniae coli of the caecum down to the base of the appendix where they converge.

If on appendicectomy a normal appendix is found, what must be ruled out?

Other causes of RIF pain (see **pain from nearby structures** above); examine the following:
1. Caecum
2. Terminal ileum (incl. Meckel's diverticulum)
3. Uterus, salpinx, ovary
4. Ureter
5. Psoas
6. Gallbladder.

Would you remove the normal appendix?

Yes (avoids confusion in diagnosis in the future).

When would you not operate?

1. If surgery is not feasible (at sea, etc)
2. If patient is a poor surgical candidate
3. If there is an appendix mass with no peritonitis.
Conservative management includes a course of antibiotics and observation. An **interval appendicectomy** can be carried out 6–8 weeks later (**Ochsner–Sherren regime**).

What is an appendix mass?

A palpable appendiceal mass with a central abscess caused by a gangrenous or perforated appendix which has become contained within omentum or loops of small bowel; abscess should be drained and interval appendicectomy performed.

What are the complications of appendicectomy?

Pre-op: perforation, peritonitis, abscess
Early post-op: wound complications (haematoma, infection) residual abscess, faecal fistula, inguinal hernia (division of ilioinguinal n.),

urinary retention, chest problems, thromboembolism.
Late post-op: adhesions.

How can they also be remembered?

***mnemonic:* WRAP IF HOT**
Wound infection
Respiratory problems (atelectasis, pneumonia)
Abscess (pelvic)
Portal pyaemia
Ileus (paralytic)
Faecal fistula
Hernia (right inguinal)
Obstruction (adhesions)
Thromboembolic phenomenon (DVT/PE).

What is Meckel's diverticulum?

A true diverticulum occurring on the **antimesenteric** border of the terminal ileum. It represents the embryological remnant of the **vitello-intestinal** duct, and has the following properties:
- Occurs in **2%** of the population
- Has a **2:1** male:female ratio
- Is approximately **2 inches** long
- Is found **2 feet** from the ileocaecal junction
- **1 in 2** will contain ectopic tissue (gastric of pancreatic)
- Only **2%** are symptomatic
- Important cause of rectal bleeding in **under 2s**

This is the **rule of 2s**.

Why does it present like an appendicitis?

If ectopic gastric mucosa present, may ulcerate and/or perforate.

How is it diagnosed?

Incidentally at operation or clinically if symptomatic. Can be scanned using IV **technetium pertechnetate** (Meckel's scan), which is preferentially taken up by gastric mucosa.

How is it treated?

Surgical excision.

CHAPTER 13: UPPER GASTROINTESTINAL BLEEDING

What is the extent of the upper GI tract?

From the pharynx to the **ligament of Trietz**.

What are the common causes of upper GI bleed?

1. Peptic ulceration (see Chapter 29b)
2. Gastritis (see Chapter 29b)
3. Oesophagitis (see Chapter 29a)
4. Oesophageal varices
5. Mallory–Weiss tear
6. Epistaxis (nosebleeds)
7. Oesophageal malignancy (see Chapter 36)
8. Gastric malignancy (see Chapter 37).

How do patients with upper GI bleed present?

Frank haematemesis: bright red blood in vomit
Coffee-ground vomit: altered blood
Melaena: black tarry stools from upper GI bleed (digested blood)
PR bleeding: a **large** upper GI bleed may present as fresh blood PR
Shock.

What is the immediate management of upper GI bleed?

1. IV access and fluids (consider CVP)
2. Oxygen
3. NGT suction (for rate and amt. of bleed)
4. Catheterise (I/O monitor)
5. Proton pump inhibitor
6. Arrange upper GI endoscopy.
If varices suspected, consider Minnesota–Sengstaken tube until endoscopy available.

What blood investigations would you do?

FBC: Hb baseline
U&Es/Cr: assess hydration and renal status

LFT: r/o liver disease (**?portal HTN** which may give rise to oesophageal varices)
Coagulation screen: r/o bleeding diatheses
GXM: this is a *must*!

What are oesophageal varices?

Dilated veins at the oesophago-gastric junction, due to porto-systemic shunting in portal hypertension.
90% due to cirrhosis in UK; worldwide, commonest cause is **schistosomiasis**.

How can you stop variceal bleeding?

Give **vasopressin** or **somatostatin**.
β-blockers also reduce portal hypertension and bleeding. Definitive intervention includes:
1. Minnesota–Sengstaken tube (if bleeding massive)
2. Endoscopic sclerotherapy or banding
3. Oesophageal transection with anastomosis (used if bleeding is refractory or recurrent)
4. Shunts: aim to shunt portal blood to caval system, hence ↓portal HTN; **TIPSS** (**T**ransjugular **I**ntrahepatic **P**orto-**S**ystemic **S**hunt) and **Warren shunt** (distal splenorenal-caval shunt). Risk of **encephalopathy** due to shunting of toxins, which are usually metabolised by the liver.

What are the poor prognostic indicators in variceal bleeding?

Age >60, jaundice, ascites, encephalopathy, hypoalbuminaemia, shock.

CHAPTER 14: OESOPHAGEAL TEARS, PERFORATION AND RUPTURE

What is Mallory–Weiss syndrome?

Longitudinal tears in the oesophageal mucosa and submucosa usually 2ry to **forceful retching** (classically after a drinking binge).

How does it present?

Haematemesis, retrosternal pain, dysphagia and odynophagia.

How is it diagnosed?

Oesophagoscopy.

What is the management?

Room temperature water lavage stops bleeding in 90% of cases. *Attempting tamponade with Minnesota–Sengstaken tube makes bleeding worse!*

What are the causes of oesophageal perforation?

Foreign body (usually sharp; most common)
Iatrogenic (eg sclerotherapy, rigid oesophagoscopy [usually at narrowest points; see Chapter 29a])
Corrosives (alkali > acid)
Carcinoma
Trauma
Infection.

What are the symptoms?

Dysphagia, odynophagia, retrosternal discomfort, dyspnoea (latter 2 from a developing **mediastinitis**).

What are the signs?

Not many, but there may be those of mediastinitis: pleural or pericardial rub, irregular pulse (arrhythmias).

What are the investigations?

ECG may show arrhythmias
CXR may show air in mediastinum (seen as black vertical shadows around cardiac silhouette)
Gastrograffin swallow: contrast seen exiting oesophagus at perforation (*don't* use barium as it may aggravate mediastinitis;

gastrograffin is water-soluble and hence safer).

What is the management?

Small perforations are usually self-resolving:
1. NBM
2. IV fluids
3. NG tube
4. PPIs
5. Regular monitoring of vitals.

Larger perforations or smaller ones which fail to resolve may require open repair.

What is oesophageal rupture known as?

Boerhaave's syndrome.

What causes it?

Trauma
Excessive vomiting (eg following a massive beer binge).

How does it present?

High mortality rate! Patient usually dead at presentation. If alive, immediate open repair is indicated, which also has a high mortality rate.

CHAPTER 15: PERFORATED PEPTIC ULCER

Which type of ulcers more commonly perforate?

Duodenal > gastric.

Which type of duodenal ulcer is more likely to perforate?

Anterior DU > Posterior DU.

What are posterior DUs more commonly associated with?

Upper GI bleeding, due to erosion of posteriorly situated gastroduodenal artery. May also cause a pancreatitis for similar reasons.

How does perforation present?

As acute upper abdominal pain which eventually becomes generalised.

What are the salient points in the history?

1. Nature of pain: typically **boring** (pt. may point to epigastrium), getting gradually worse and more generalised
2. Associated vomiting and malaise
3. History of PUD (50% have none) or ZES
4. Medications: NSAIDs and steroids (can cause ulcers)
5. Ulcer surgery in past.

What are the relevant clinical findings?

General: Ill-looking patient, lying still; may be Cushingoid 2ry to steroid use
Hands: Cool and clammy; tachycardic
Abdomen: Peritonitic. Not moving with respiration, tender generally, but maximally in epigastrium; rebound and guarding; reduced bowel sounds; tympany over liver.

What are the differentials?

1. Acute pancreatitis
2. Acute cholecystitis
3. Other perforated viscus (eg diverticulae)
4. Acute MI.

What investigations would you do?

Blood investigations:
1. FBC: Hb as pt. will need a laparotomy; ↑WBC in peritonitis

2. U+Es: may be altered 2ry to vomiting
3. Amylase: r/o pancreatitis (though may be slightly raised in perforated ulcer)
4. LFTs: r/o cholecystitis
5. G&S: for operation.

Radiology: erect CXR for free air under diaphragm (80% of time).

Other: ECG to r/o acute MI.

What is your management?

1. Admit to ward
2. NBM
3. NGT ($\downarrow$peritoneal cavity contamination)
4. IVF + correct electrolyte imbalance (K^+, etc.)
5. Catheterise and I/O charting
6. Antibiotics (eg cefuroxime + metronidazole)
7. Analgesia (opioids)
8. Consent for laparotomy +/− proceed.

What else should you arrange?

Possible ITU bed post-operatively, especially in patients with co-morbidities (eg COPD).

What operation would you do?

Exploratory laparotomy and either simple closure of the ulcer by edge apposition, or by use of an omental patch (Graham patch). Follow this by **copious irrigation** of peritoneal cavity with warm saline.

What about a definitive procedure?

Pt. will need one (if fit) to prevent recurrence. Type of operation dependent on whether ulcer is gastric or duodenal (see Chapter 29b).

When is conservative management advised?

In patients unfit for anaesthesia. Management is otherwise as above with continual re-assessment.

CHAPTER 16: CHOLECYSTITIS, CHOLANGITIS AND EMPYEMA OF THE GALLBLADDER

ACUTE CHOLECYSTITIS

What is acute cholecystitis?

Acute inflammation of the gallbladder.

What is the pathogenesis?

Obstruction of the cystic duct leading to inflammation. 95% caused by gallstones (see Chapter 29e); 5% to calculus obstruction.

How does it present?

1. Constant RUQ pain, referred to epigastrium and to right scapular tip (**Boas' sign**)
2. Fever (24–36 h after pain), nausea and vomiting
3. May give a history of gallstones: RUQ discomfort, especially after greasy meal; jaundice/dark urine/pale stools
4. Pt. may have already been diagnosed and is awaiting cholecystectomy.

What are the clinical findings?

General: Ill-looking patient in pain
Hands: Sweaty palms, tachycardia
Abdomen: Tenderness in RUQ +/– epigastrium; positive **Murphy's sign** (see p. 23).

What are the differentials?

1. Peptic ulcer disease
2. Acute pancreatitis
3. Acute MI.

What investigations would you do?

Blood investigations:
1. FBC: ↑WBC
2. U+Es: Electrolyte disturbance in vomiting
3. LFTs: ↑ALP in biliary tree disease; ↑bilirubin in obstructive jaundice

4. Amylase: r/o pancreatitis (though may be mildly raised in cholecystitis)

Radiology: USS (test of choice)

Other: ECG (if pt. is high-risk for MI).

What's the management?

1. Admit to ward
2. NBM
3. IVF and correct electrolyte imbalance
4. IV antibiotics (broad spectrum)
5. Opiate analgesia
6. Elective cholecystectomy in 6 weeks.

What are the complications?

1. Empyema (abscess of the gallbladder)
2. Gallbladder perforation with bile peritonitis
3. Obstructive jaundice due to:
   a. Stone passing into CBD
   b. CBD obstruction 2ry to local oedema (inflamed gallbladder pressing on nearby CBD)
4. Cholecystenteric fistula (between gallbladder and small bowel) and gallstone ileus (see Chapter 18).

Why do a cholecystectomy?

Because of high risk of a recurrent attack and its associated complications.

Why in 6 weeks time?

Local oedema and distortion of tissue planes makes an emergency cholecystectomy technically more difficult with an increased risk of gallbladder perforation (inflamed gallbladder is **friable**).

Is there *ever* an indication for operating in the acute setting?

1. Failure of conservative management (10%)
2. Development of the complications above

What is it?

A severe infection complicating distal CBD obstruction, spreading proximally. Syn: **ascending cholangitis.**

What organisms are involved?

Usually Gram –ve bacilli (*E. coli*, *Klebsiella*, *Enterobacter*, *Proteus*, *Serratia*)

How does it present?

Classically with **Charcot's triad:**
1. Fever with rigors
2. Jaundice
3. RUQ pain.

In severe infection, there may be added **sepsis** and **alterations in CNS status**, all 5 symptoms constituting **Reynold's pentad** (see p. 24).

What investigations would you do?

Blood investigations:
1. FBC: ↑WBC
2. U+Es: Electrolyte disturbance in vomiting
3. LFTs: ↑ALP in biliary tree disease; ↑bilirubin in obstructive jaundice
4. Blood cultures: r/o sepsis.

Radiology: USS is the investigation of choice.

What is the management?

This is a surgical emergency as **endotoxic shock** may ensue.
1. Admit to ward
2. NBM
3. IVF and correct electrolyte imbalance
4. IV antibiotics (directed towards coliforms) eg cefuroxime, gentamicin and metronidazole
5. Opioids
6. Emergency ERCP with stone extraction once clinically stable.

What are the complications?

1. Endotoxic shock
2. Suppurative cholangitis (pus in biliary tree).

| Are there any indications for operating in cholangitis? | Generally no (hazardous), except in **suppurative cholangitis:** laparotomy with T-tube insertion to drain pus (done only if ERCP and PTC drainage have failed). |

EMPYEMA

What is an empyema?	A pus-filled gallbladder.
What are the causes?	1. Severe acute cholecystitis (2–3% of cases) 2. Super-infected mucocoele.
What is a mucocoele?	Mucus-filled gallbladder; caused by impaction of a gallstone at the gallbladder neck. This results in stasis. Continued mucus production results in its build-up.
How does empyema present?	Malaise, nausea/vomiting, **swinging pyrexia**.
What are the investigations?	**Blood investigations:** 1. FBC: ↑WBC 2. Blood cultures: r/o sepsis.
How would you treat it?	This is a surgical emergency (25% mortality) 1. Admit 2. NBM 3. IVF and correct electrolyte imbalance 4. IV antibiotics (cef/gent/metro) 5. Opioids 6. Drainage via percutaneous placement of a **pigtail catheter** into the gallbladder (USS or CT-guided).
Would you operate?	Only if radiological catheter placement has failed. Operation: open I&D of empyema +/− cholecystectomy.

CHAPTER 17: PANCREATITIS

APPLIED ANATOMY

Where is the pancreas located?	In the retroperitoneum, forming part of the stomach bed.
What are its parts?	Head, uncinate process, neck, body, and tail.
What is its blood supply?	Mainly from the splenic a., but also contributions from the sup. and inf. pancreaticoduodenal aa. (head); venous drainage via splenic v. (drains into portal v.)
What are its functions?	It is both an exocrine and endocrine gland. ***Exocrine:*** produces pancreatic juice containing **trypsin**, **lipase**, and **amylase** (acinar glands) which aids in digestion. ***Endocrine:*** produces glucagon (α-cells) and insulin (β-cells) from the islets of Langerhans located in the tail.

ACUTE PANCREATITIS

What is acute pancreatitis?	Acute inflammation of the pancreas characterised by sudden onset of abdominal pain and raised pancreatic enzymes in the blood and urine. It may recur.
What occurs during pancreatitis?	There is autodigestion of pancreatic tissue by its own enzymes.
What are the causes of pancreatitis?	***mnemonic:* GET SMASHED** **G**allstones (most common cause in UK) **E**thanol **T**rauma **S**teroids **M**umps (also Coxsackie)

Autoimmune (polyarteritis nodosa)
Scorpion bite (common in Trinidad; South American black-bellied variety)
Hypercalcaemia, **H**ypothermia, **H**yperlipidaemia
ERCP, **E**mboli
Drugs (thiazides, azathioprine, oestrogens).

Often no cause is found; gallstones and ethanol account for 80% in UK.

How does acute pancreatitis present?

Epigastric pain typically boring through to back and relieved by **leaning forward**. If severe, pain may be widespread.
Nausea and vomiting +/− fever
Varying consciousness (symptoms of shock).

What are the important points to note in the history?

1. Age of patient (important in Ranson's criteria)
2. Elucidate a cause (see above) as this may alter long-term management (eg ERCP/cholecystectomy in gallstones; Pabrinex in alcoholics)
3. Prior episodes (1st episode or acute on chronic pancreatitis?)
4. Symptoms suggestive of differential diagnoses.

What are the clinical findings?

General: Ill-looking patient, possibly sweating and confused if shocked
Hands: Cool, clammy peripheries; tachycardic
Abdomen: Tender with localised rebound tenderness (generalised if peritonitic); possible bowel sounds (paralytic ileus); possible mass (pseudocyst, sentinel loop).

What clinical signs do you know of?	**Grey Turner's sign, Cullen's sign** and **Fox's sign** (see pp. 21, 22). These are signs of **retroperitoneal haemorrhage**, a sign of **haemorrhagic pancreatitis** (see below).
What are the differential diagnoses?	Gastritis/PUD Acute cholecystitis Peritonitis (2ry to perforated viscus) High intestinal obstruction MI.
Do you know of a scoring system used to grade the prognosis of pancreatitis?	**Ranson's criteria**: *mnemonic:* Criteria at presentation: **GA LAW** (*Georgia Law*) **G**lucose >10 mmol/L (pt not diabetic) **A**ge >55 (or >70 if gallstones) **L**DH >350 i.u./L **A**ST >250 i.u./L **W**BC >16,000 (10^9/L. Criteria during next 48 hours: **COUCH** **C**alcium < 2.0 mmol/L (corrected) **O**xygen (PO_2) < 8 kPa **U**rea increase > 10 mmol/L despite IV fluids **C**oncealed (ie estimated sequestered) fluid > 6 L **H**aematocrit increase > 10%. 1 point is given for each criterion present; severe pancreatitis = 3 or more points.
What blood tests should be ordered?	Based on the criteria above, the following bloods should be ordered: 1. **FBC**: WBC and Hct; also Hb if bleeding suspected 2. **U+Es**: urea; also reflects state of hydration 3. **LFTs**: AST, LDH; raised ALP suggests gallstones as a cause

4. **Bone profile**: calcium
5. **Random blood sugar**
6. **ABG**: PO_2; also metabolic acidosis
7. **Amylase**: **not one of the criteria,** but becomes markedly raised in pancreatitis and aids in diagnosis
8. **GXM** if haemorrhage and shock are suspected
9. **CRP** as a baseline (an **independent criterion** of prognosis); serial CRPs are used to monitor response to treatment
10. **Lipid profile** to rule out hyperlipidaemia as cause.

What else can give a raised amylase?

mnemonic: **AMYLASE**
AAA rupture
Mesenteric ischaemia
g**Y**nae pathology (ovarian tumour)
Liver disease
Anuria (renal failure)
Salivary gland disease (tumour, inflammation)/**S**tomach ulcer (perforated)
Ectopic pregnancy (also DKA).

What other investigations should be performed?

On admission:
1. **Erect CXR**: look for air under diaphragm to r/o perforated DU, and for pleural effusion/ARDS (cotton wool opacification throughout lung fields).
2. **AXR**: **sentinel loop** (most common sign on AXR), gallstones (only 10% visible), calcific stippling (saponification seen in chronic pancreatitis; rare).

Subsequently:

3. **USS**: gallstones, pseudocyst, abscess, necrosis
4. **CT**: if pseudocyst, abscess or necrosis suspected
5. **ERCP**: if cholelithiasis suspected.

What is the treatment?

1. Admit to ward (ITU if severe)
2. IV fluids
3. NBM
4. Catheterise and I/O charting
5. NGT
6. PCA
7. PPIs
8. IV antibiotics (moderate to severe only)
9. Insulin sliding scale (if blood sugar high).

How can this be remembered?

mnemonic: **PANCREAS**

PPIs
Analgesia (PCA)
NBM
Catheterise
Rehydrate (IV fluids)
Empty stomach (NGT)
Antibiotics (severe only)
Sliding scale insulin (if blood sugar high).

What are the complications?

mnemonic: **PANCREAS!**

Pseudocyst/**P**hlegmon
Airway problems (**A**RDS, pleural effusion), **A**scites
Necrosis (may lead to haemorrhagic pancreatitis)/Abscess
Coagulation disorder/DIC; **C**alcium deficit
Renal failure/MOF
Encephalopathy
Arterial (splenic/mesenteric/portal vessel rupture or thrombosis)
Sugar (diabetes); **S**IRS; **S**epsis.

What is a pseudocyst?

An encapsulated collection of pancreatic fluid and necrotic material which usually collects in the **lesser sac** (between the pancreas and posterior wall of stomach). Usually occurs in **chronic alcoholic pancreatitis** after 2nd week (1–8%)
Symptoms: same as pancreatitis; suspect in a patient with acute pancreatitis whose pain does not resolve
Signs: palpable, tender epigastric mass
Investigations: amylase (persistently elevated); USS abdomen
Treatment: depends on size (controversial); If <5 cm, close follow-up to see if resolving If >5 cm, either percutaneous USS-guided aspiration or surgical **marsupialisation** of pseudocyst into posterior wall of stomach (**cystogastrostomy**).

What is a pancreatic abscess?

A collection of purulent peri-pancreatic fluid
Symptoms: swinging pyrexia and continuing malaise.
Signs: palpable, tender, epigastric mass
Investigations: USS abdomen/CT scan
Treatment: either CT-guided needle aspiration or open I+D; broad spectrum IV antibiotics.

What is pancreatic necrosis?

Dead pancreatic tissue following acute pancreatitis. Presents in a similar manner to pancreatic abscess.
Investigations: CT scan with IV contrast; dead tissue doesn't take contrast up
Treatment: surgical debridement.

What is haemorrhagic pancreatitis?	Retroperitoneal bleeding secondary to extensive pancreatic necrosis. **Symptoms:** shock, abdominal pain, respiratory distress (2ry to ARDS) **Signs:** Grey Turner's, Cullen's, Fox's (see above) **Investigations:** ↑amylase, ↓Hct, ↓Ca^{2+}; CT scan with IV contrast **Treatment:** supportive.

CHRONIC PANCREATITIS

What is chronic pancreatitis?	Chronic pancreatitis is a continuing inflammatory process characterised by irreversible morphological change, pain +/− loss of function.
What are the causes?	As for acute pancreatitis, but alcohol is most common.
How does it present?	Epigastric pain which is unremitting; weight loss; steatorrhoea.
How does functional loss present?	**Exocrine:** ↓lipase = fat malabsorption = *steatorrhoea* **Endocrine:** ↓insulin = glucose intolerance = *diabetes*.
What investigations should be performed?	Blood investigations as with acute pancreatitis.
Is amylase also raised in chronic pancreatitis?	It can be, but may be normal due to 'pancreatic burn-out' (extensive tissue loss).
Any other investigations?	AXR: calcific stippling (saponification; rare) USS/CT scan: gland enlargement or atrophy.
What are the treatment options?	**Conservative:** 1. Stop alcohol (AA if necessary) 2. Treat IDDM 3. Narcotics 4. Pancreatic enzyme replacement.

Surgical:
1. Removal of pancreatic duct stones
2. Partial pancreatectomy of body and tail (duct stenosis)
3. Sphincteroplasty of pancreatic duct opening
4. Total pancreatectomy.

CHAPTER 18: BOWEL OBSTRUCTION

What types of obstruction do you know of?

Mechanical obstruction (small and large bowel obstruction) and **functional obstruction** (paralytic ileus and pseudo-obstruction).

MECHANICAL OBSTRUCTION

What is the natural course of mechanical obstruction (pathophysiology)?

Bowel dilation proximal to the obstruction
- Intraluminal gas and fluid accumulation (**fluid sequestration** or **'third space loss'**) and resultant **dehydration**
- Bowel wall **oedema** 2ry to dilation
- Arterial and venous blood flow impairment 2ry to oedema, leading to bowel wall **ischaemia** (known as **bowel strangulation**)
- **Infarction** and **perforation** of affected bowel segment 2ry to ischaemia, with spillage of bowel contents into peritoneum
- Continuing dehydration, peritonitis, electrolyte imbalance and systemic toxicity.

What are the causes?

(See Table 18.1; most common causes are highlighted **bold**)

What are the cardinal features of mechanical obstruction?

1. Colicky abdominal pain
2. Abdominal distension
3. Vomiting
4. Obstipation.

So do small and large bowel obstruction present in the same way, then?

No, the timing of each symptom varies depending on the type and level of obstruction (see Table 18.2).

Is the nature of the vomit important?

Yes; gives a rough indication of duration of obstruction:
Early: gastric and small intestinal contents

Table 18.1

	Small bowel	Large bowel
Extraluminal	• **Adhesions (60%)** • **Malignancy (20%)** • **Herniae (10%)** • Volvulus • Intussusception • Congenital bands	• **Volvulus (15%)** • Malignancy • Intussusception
Mural	• **Crohn's (5%)** • Carcinoma • TB • Congenital atresia	• **Carcinoma (50%)** • **Diverticular disease (10%)** • TB
Luminal	• Gallstones (see below) • Polypoid tumours • Bezoars • Foreign bodies • Parasites	• Faecal impaction • Polypoid tumours • Parasites

Table 18.2

	Small bowel	Large bowel
Colicky abdominal pain	Mainly central (midgut structure)	Mainly suprapubic (hindgut structure)
Abdominal distension	Present to a lesser degree	More pronounced
Vomiting	Occurs early	Occurs late
Obstipation	Occurs late; pt. may pass some initial flatus and faeces	Occurs early, usually with complete obstipation (but may be partial)

Late: Faeculent due to stagnation and intestinal overgrowth (usually **effortless** by this stage).

Can it present in any other way?

Yes. There may be a history of:
1. Fever and malaise: suggests infarction/perforation/peritonitis
2. Thirst and lethargy: dehydration from 3rd space loss or sepsis.

The patient may also present in septic shock.

What are the other important points in the history?

1. History of colorectal disease (carcinoma, diverticular disease), herniae, SBO in past or gallstones (gallstone ileus)
2. Surgical history, including post-surgery radiotherapy in carcinoma (adhesions).

What are the clinical features?

General: Pt. in pain, actively vomiting
Hands: Febrile and tachycardic in ischaemia/peritonitis
Abdomen: Distended abdomen +/– visible peristalsis; tender centrally on palpation +/– rebound (if peritonitic). **Tympany** on percussion. **Tinkling (high pitched) bowel sounds** (may be **reduced** in ischaemia).

What *must* you rule out on examination?

1. Herniae (examine groins, umbilicus, epigastrium and scars) (see Chapter 28)
2. Anorectal pathology (perform a DRE).

What are the investigations?

Blood investigations:
1. FBC: ↓Hb (malignancy, ?fit for surgery), ↑WBC (infarction, perforation)
2. U+Es: Electrolyte disturbance (sequestration, vomiting)
3. Amylase: r/o pancreatitis in an acute abdomen
4. G&S: may need surgery
5. ABG: if ischaemia suspected (**metabolic acidosis**).
Radiology: see individual management below.

What are the radiological investigations?

Plain films: CXR to r/o visceral perforation; **AXR** shows the following features:
- **Central** dilated bowel loops
- **Valvulae conniventes** (bands which **fully traverse** the bowel diameter)
- Dilation of **>5 cm** (pathological).

Double-contrast CT scan: in stable patients only where urgent surgery is not indicated. Shows:
- Level of obstruction
- Cause of obstruction
- Bowel viability.

What is the initial management?

Conservative ('drip and suck' regime):
1. Admit
2. NBM
3. IVF (**drip**) and correct electrolyte disturbances
4. NGT (**suck**) to decompress **stomach**, *not* bowel (prevents aspiration)
5. Urinary catheter
6. Oxygen
7. Opioids
8. Vitals 2-hourly.

How would you follow this patient?

With 8-hourly abdominal examinations.

When would you abandon conservative management?

- If signs of **bowel strangulation** ensue:
  1. Tachycardia
  2. Fever
  3. Localised tenderness and peritonism; if conservative management **fails**; in the presence of an **irreducible hernia**.

What surgery would you do?	Exploratory laparotomy.
Why?	To achieve the following: 1. Decompress bowel 2. Correct cause 3. Resect non-viable bowel 4. Maintain bowel continuity (if possible).
How would you assess bowel viability at laparotomy?	In the affected segment, assess the following: 1. **Colour:** green/black = non-viable; plum = wrap in warm saline-soaked pack for few minutes and re-assess for peristalsis 2. **Sheen:** absence = non-viable 3. **Peristalsis:** absence = non-viability 4. **Mesenteric pulsatility:** absence = non-viability.
If bowel is resected, would you directly anastomose the ends or fashion a stoma?	(See Chapter 3 on anastomoses and stomas)
How should the bowel be handled at laparotomy?	*As little as possible:* prevents **paralytic ileus** post-operatively (see below).
What are the complications of extensive bowel resection?	These mainly arise from insufficient absorption of: 1. Vitamins (see Chapter 5 for vitamin deficiencies) 2. Fats, causing steatorrhoea or diarrhoea 3. Calcium, causing osteoporosis.

MANAGEMENT OF LARGE BOWEL OBSTRUCTION (LBO)

What are the radiological investigations?	**Plain films: CXR** to r/o visceral perforation **AXR** shows the following features: • **Peripheral** dilated bowel loops • **Haustrae** (bands which

incompletely traverse the bowel diameter)
- Dilation of **>8 cm** (pathological, **>10 cm** in **caecal dilation**)

In stable patients not requiring urgent surgical intervention, the following can be used:
- **Double-contract Ba enema:** shows level of obstruction but not cause. *Do not use in complete obstruction due to* **risk of perforation**. Instead, use **single-contrast, gastrograffin enema** (water-soluble, so no peritonitis if perforation occurs)
- **Double-contrast CT abdomen:** (see above).

What is the difference between single- and double-contrast barium enema?

Single-contrast uses Ba only. **Double-contrast** uses Ba administered with **air**, hence giving superior anatomical detail on imaging. In complete obstruction, air may precipitate perforation 2ry to dilation.

What is the significance of caecal dilation on the film?

'The caecum bears the brunt of large bowel obstruction.' In complete obstruction, caecum dilates and may even present as a **RIF mass**. Perforation occurs here first. Pathological caecal dilation is an indication for surgery.

Which patients are especially at risk of caecal dilation?

Those with a **competent ileocaecal valve**, a valve between the caecum and terminal ileum which prevents bowel content **backflow**. Increased pressure in caecum has no outlet to 'vent' through.

How would you assess ileocaecal competence on the plain film?

An incompetent valve will show up as both large *and* small bowel obstruction as increased pressure 'vents' backwards through valve into the terminal ileum.

What is the management?	**'Drip and suck regime'** (see p. 161). Consent for laparotomy.
Why is a trial of conservatism not attempted first?	Large bowel blood supply is more tenuous than small bowel, therefore greater risk of **bowel wall ischaemia**.
What are the principles of surgery in large bowel obstruction?	Same as for small bowel obstruction (see above).
What *must* be ruled out before considering surgery?	Pseudo-obstruction (see below).

FUNCTIONAL OBSTRUCTION

What types do you know of?	Paralytic ileus and pseudo-obstruction
What are the causes of functional obstruction?	*mnemonic:* **CRAMPED** (think of dilated loops of bowel cramped-up in the abdominal cavity): **C**VA **R**enal failure, **R**etroperitoneal haemorrhage **A**bdominal malignancy **M**I, **M**yxoedema, **M**esenteric vascular disease **P**ost-operative, **P**neumonia, **P**eritonitis, **P**elvic abscess **E**lectrolyte disturbance **D**amaged bones (orthopaedic trauma, incl. spinal and head injury), **D**rugs (tricyclic antidepressants, GA), **D**KA.

PARALYTIC ILEUS

What is it?	Massive **non-obstructive small bowel** dilation.
How does it present?	Similar to small bowel obstruction, but with important differences: paralytic ileus is usually **silent** and **painless**. The most common cause is **post-operative**.
What are the investigations?	As with SBO (see above). **Gastrograffin study** can be done in addition to plain film if doubt exists as to whether obstruction is functional or mechanical.
What is the management?	**Conservative** ('drip and suck'; see above). No place for surgery. Usually resolves in 4–5 days.

PSEUDO-OBSTRUCTION

What is it?	Massive **non-obstructive colonic** dilation.
How does it present?	Like large bowel obstruction but with reduced colonic motility (↓ bowel sounds).
What are the investigations?	Do a **single-contrast gastrograffin enema** to r/o a lesion causing mechanical obstruction.
How is it managed?	Conservatively, including removal of precipitating factor. Surgery for decompression only if this fails (**tube caecostomy** or **resection**).

SPECIFIC CAUSES OF BOWEL OBSTRUCTION

VOLVULUS

What is it?	Twisting of the colon about its mesenteric pedicle resulting in **mechanical obstruction**.
What types do you know of?	**Sigmoid** and **caecal** volvulus.
What is the big risk of volvulus?	**Bowel infarction** and its associated risks due to vascular compromise at the twisted pedicle.
How does it present?	As mechanical large bowel obstruction (see above).
How do the two types compare?	(See Table 18.3).

GALLSTONE ILEUS

What is it?	SBO caused by large intraluminal gallstone.
How does it happen?	Gallbladder with large gallstone lies against small bowel • Gallstone erodes through the walls of both to lie in small bowel lumen, thus creating a **cholecystoenteric fistula** • Descends down small bowel and causes obstruction, usually at **ileocaecal valve.** Can also happen post-endoscopic sphincterotomy.
How common is it?	Accounts for <1% of all obstructions, ie **rare**! (If asked the causes of SBO, *don't say this first!*)
Who gets it?	Most common in elderly females (though still rare).

Table 18.3

	Sigmoid volvulus	Caecal volvulus
Incidence	75% of all volvulus cases	25% of all volvulus cases
Aetiology	• High residue diet (↑ in Africa) • Laxative abuse • Pregnancy • Prior abdominal Sx • Bed-ridden	Poor fixation of caecum during previous surgery
Radiological findings	• **Plain film:** grossly dilated sigmoid colon giving **bent inner-tube** or **omega** sign • **Contrast study:** if diagnosis unsure; gives **bird-beak** appearance	• **Plain film:** grossly dilated caecum giving **coffee-bean** sign. • **Contrast study:** if diagnosis unsure.
Treatment	• **Conservative: sigmoidoscopy** may reduce volvulus (80%; also diagnostic); if not, try **Ba enema**. • **Surgical:** if conservative fails, or in strangulation; do reduction +/– bowel resection + stoma formation if strangulation present	• **Surgical:** emergency **caecopexy**; right hemicolectomy if infarction present +/– stoma. (No place for conservative management)

What are the classical X-ray findings?

1. Dilated loops of small bowel
2. Radio-opaque gallstone distal to obstruction, usually at ileocaecal junction (RIF)
3. Air in biliary tree (**air cholecystogram**); seen in 40% of cases and is due to cholecystoenteric fistula.

CT scan shows the same findings.

What is the treatment?

Laparotomy with **enterotomy** and stone removal +/– either cholecystoenteric fistula repair or cholecystectomy.

What other cause of a cholecystoenteric fistula do you know of?

Gallbladder cancer (see Chapter 42).

CHAPTER 19: DIVERTICULAR DISEASE

What is diverticulosis?
The **incidental** presence of diverticulae (sing. diverticulum) in the colon.

What are these diverticulae?
Small out-pouchings from the wall of the colon.

Are they true diverticulae?
No, they are **pseudo-diverticulae**, as their wall does not comprise all the layers of the bowel wall. They are actually **mucosal out-pouchings** which occur at areas of weakness in the bowel wall.

Give an example of a true diverticulum.
Meckel's diverticulum (see Chapter 12).

Where are these areas of weakness in the bowel wall?
At the points of entry of blood vessels into the bowel wall.

So what causes these out-pouchings to occur?
Increased intraluminal pressure caused by **low-fibre diets** (the bowel has to work harder to push low-residue, low-bulk stool through).

What is the incidence of diverticulosis?
1/3 of the population in the Western world has **diverticulosis** by age 60 years.

Which part of the bowel is most affected?
The **sigmoid colon**, although the entire colon can be affected.

Do diverticulae have any malignant potential?
No.

How does it present?
Mainly asymptomatic, being picked up incidentally on imaging for other causes, but can present as vague LIF/suprapubic pain, diarrhoea and flatulence. It may also present as one of the complications of diverticular disease.

What are these complications?	1. Diverticulitis 2. Diverticular bleed (see Chapter 21).
How is uncomplicated diverticulosis diagnosed?	Barium enema (test of choice): diverticulae are clearly defined by barium. CT scan will also show diverticulae.
What about colonoscopy?	Not ideal; diverticulae are difficult to visualise.
How is uncomplicated diverticulosis treated?	With a **high-fibre diet**.
What about surgery?	Surgery as a 1-stage resection of the affected segment and re-anastomosis of the bowel can be considered in those cases who have symptoms not relieved by conservative measures, or those who have recurrent flare-up of complications.
What is diverticulitis?	Inflammation of 1 or more diverticulae.
How does it present?	Fever, malaise, n/v, LIF pain +/– diarrhoea. Dysuria if inflamed diverticulum rests on ureter/bladder.
What are the clinical findings?	*General:* ill-looking, sweating, febrile *Hands:* tachycardia *Abdomen:* localised rebound and guarding in the LIF *DRE:* normal.
Based on the history and examination, what is diverticulitis sometimes known as?	Left-sided appendicitis.
What are the investigations?	**Blood investigations:** leucocytosis. **Imaging: AXR** may show partially obstructed bowel; **CXR** may show air under diaphragm if perforation of inflamed diverticulum has occurred.

Would you do a barium enema?	No! Risk of perforation in inflamed bowel.
What about colonoscopy?	Again, no! Spasm of inflamed bowel may cause perforation.
What complications of diverticulitis can occur?	1. Diverticular abscess 2. Perforation with resultant peritonitis 3. Fistula 4. Stenosis with resultant obstruction.
How would you manage it?	**Uncomplicated** diverticulitis is managed as follows: 1. Admit 2. IV fluids 3. IV cef/gent/metro (check local policy) 4. Analgesia 5. Observe for complications 6. Regular vitals. Most cases will settle with this.
What about the complications?	**Diverticular abscess:** collection of pus locally occurring around an inflamed diverticulum. *Clinical:* localised abdominal pain, malaise, n/v, swinging pyrexia and rigors. *Investigations:* CT abdomen shows abscess *Treatment:* antibiotics; CT-guided aspiration or open surgical drainage if former fails. **Perforation:** inflamed diverticulum perforates, releasing faeculent matter into peritoneum. Peritonitis ensues. *Clinical:* fever, malaise, n/v, peritonitic abdomen (board-like rigidity, generalised rebound and guarding, absent bowel sounds) *Investigations:* CXR shows free air

under diaphragm; CT scan may show location

Treatment: antibiotics and laparotomy with resection of involved segment of colon and stoma formation (eg Hartmann's procedure) and re-joining at a later date (see Chapter 3).

Fistula: caused by inflamed tip of diverticulum eroding into nearby structure. Examples are:

• Colovesical (bowel to bladder)
• Colovaginal (bowel to vagina)

Clinical: will depend on type of fistula:

• Colovesical: pneumaturia, recurrent UTIs
• Colovaginal: faeculent vaginal discharge

Investigations: CT scan or fistulogram
Treatment: see Chapter 3.

Stenosis: caused by repeated diverticulitis causing scarring. Large bowel obstruction may ensue (see Chapter 18). Stenotic colon 2ry to diverticular disease may look identical to carcinoma, which must be ruled out. The stenotic segment may need to be resected.

Can bleeding occur during diverticulitis?

Yes, but it is *unusual*. Diverticular bleed occurs as a separate entity (see Chapter 21).

CHAPTER 20: INFLAMMATORY BOWEL DISEASE: ULCERATIVE COLITIS AND CROHN'S DISEASE

What are the differences between Crohn's disease (CD) and ulcerative colitis (UC)?

See Table 20.1

Table 20.1

	Crohn's disease (CD)	Ulcerative colitis (UC)
Definition	**Regional enteritis** affecting any part of the bowel from mouth to anus. **Rectal sparing** seen	Enteritis of the large bowel only, with **anal sparing**
Incidence	6:100,000 (bimodal; ie 2 peaks in lifetime incidence); High in Jewish population, low in Afro-Caribbean	26:100,000 (bimodal); High in Jewish population, low in Afro-Caribbean
Age	25–40, then 50–65	20–35, then 50–65
Sex	F > M	F = M
Geography	More common in developing countries	More common in developing countries
Aetiology	?Autoimmune; environmental factors postulated	?Autoimmune; environmental factors postulated
Pathology	*Microscopic:* **Non-caseating granulomas**; Full thickness (**transmural**) involvement; Transverse fissures; Crypt distortion; Deep ulcers	*Microscopic:* Musosal/submucosal involvement only; Metaplasia and dysplasia; Flat, granular mucosa; **Crypt abscesses**; Shallow ulcers

Table 20.1 (continued)

	Crohn's disease (CD)	Ulcerative colitis (UC)
	Gross: Swollen mucosa (**cobblestone appearance**); **Skip lesions**; Mouth to anus affected (but rectal involvement rare); Serosal **fat encroachment**; Fibrosis and strictures	*Gross:* **Pseudopolyps**; Only colon and rectum affected (occasionally terminal ileum: **'backwash ileitis'**); Normal serosa (except in toxic megacolon)
Presentation	*General:* Malaise, weight loss, anorexia *Intestinal:* Mostly **anal**: fissure, ulceration, fistulae (multiple perianal fistulae leads to **watering-can perineum**) Also, colitis: bloody diarrhoea with **mucus** Fibrosis and **stricture** formation may lead to **chronic obstruction** Isolated **terminal ileitis** may mimic appendicitis Other fistulae: enterocutaneous, enterocystic, enterovaginal *Extraintestinal:* See below	*General:* Malaise, weight loss, anorexia *Intestinal:* Mostly **colorectal**: urgent defecation with **bleeding** and **mucus** due to **colitis** (hallmark of UC) Constipation in **proctitis** Massive colonic distension and resulting sepsis in **toxic megacolon** (colonic diameter >6 cm on plain film) Risk of **cancer** (2% at 10 years, then ↑ by 2% yearly after that) *Extraintestinal:* See below

Table 20.1 (continued)

	Crohn's disease (CD)	Ulcerative colitis (UC)
Investigations	*Blood investigations:* FBC: anaemia, ↑WBC ↑ESR and CRP (acute phase) ↓albumin (acute)	*Blood investigations:* FBC: anaemia, ↑WBC ↑ESR and CRP (acute phase) ↓albumin (acute)
	Imaging: Ba studies: skip lesions, cobblestone appearance, fistulae, '**rosethorn' ulcers** and **Kantor's string sign** (narrowed bowel segments with proximal dilation)	*Imaging:* Ba studies: affected rectum with proximal, continuous spread; pseudopolyps, uniform **hosepipe colon** (2ry to ↓ haustrae)
	Endoscopy: As above. Useful for assessing disease distribution and taking biopsies	*Endoscopy:* As with Crohn's disease
	Stool cultures: Rule out infective colitis	*Stool cultures:* Rule out infective colitis
	Resuscitate with IV fluids	Resuscitate with IV fluids
Management	*Medical:* 1. Anti-inflammatories: oral 5′-aminosalicyclic acid (5′-ASA) preparations (eg sulphasalazine, mesalazine) 2. Steroids (eg prednisolone) 3. Antibiotics: metronidazole is usually reserved for complications such as perianal disease in CD	*Medical:* As with Crohn's disease

Table 20.1 (continued)

	Crohn's disease (CD)	Ulcerative colitis (UC)
	1 and 2 can also both be used topically as foam enemas	
	Surgical: **Not curative** Reserved for failure of medical management or complications of CD (eg fistulae, perforation)	*Surgical:* **Curative** Reserved for failure of medical management; pts. with high risk of malignancy (early onset UC) or malignancy on biopsy; or complications of UC (eg toxic megacolon, severe haemorrhage)
	Should be as **conservative and limited** as possible. High risk of post-op sepsis and further fistulae. **Multiple laparotomies** are common for segmental bowel resections, stricturoplasty and fistula resection	Should be **radical**. Removal of diseased segment may cure patient (low risk of recurrence). In emergency situation, perform **subtotal colectomy** and **ileostomy**. Elective **panproctocolectomy** is performed if entire bowel is affected by UC, or pre-malignant changes have occurred

What are the extraintestinal manifestations of IBD?

Many! Being systematic will help: examine skin, hands, face (eyes then mouth), abdomen and musculoskeletal.

Skin: erythema nodosum, pyoderma gangrenosum

Hands: digital clubbing

Face: Eyes: iritis; *Mouth:* aphthous ulcers

Abdomen: mainly **hepatobiliary** (chronic active hepatitis, cirrhosis, sclerosing cholangitis, biliary duct carcinoma) and **renal** (amyloidosis and nephrotic syndrome)

Musculoskeletal: large joint arthritis, ankylosing spondylitis, sacroiliitis.

CHAPTER 21: LOWER GASTROINTESTINAL BLEEDING

What is the extent of the lower GI tract?

From the **ligament of Trietz** to the anus.

What are the causes of lower GI bleeding?

Altered blood:
1. Upper GI bleed
2. Right-sided colon neoplasm (see Chapter 39)

Fresh blood:
1. Haemorrhoids (see Chapter 30b)
2. Diverticular disease (see Chapter 19)
3. Left sided colon neoplasm (see Chapter 39)
4. Inflammatory bowel disease (see Chapter 20)
5. Angiodysplasia
6. Ischaemic bowel
7. Pseudomembranous colitis
8. Infective causes eg salmonella.

What are the important points in the history?

Is the blood bright red or dark/altered?
- Distinguishes left and right sided colonic pathology

Is the blood mixed with the stool?
- Suggests malignancy

Is the blood in the toilet pan or on the paper?
- In pan suggests diverticular disease; on paper suggests anal pathology (haemorrhoids/fissure)

Any recent change in bowel habit?
- Again, suggests malignancy

Is there any family history of bowel disease?
- Carcinoma and IBD have a familial tendency.

What is your immediate management?

1. Admit
2. IVF and correct electrolyte imbalance
3. Catheterise; I/O monitor (if bleeding brisk).

What investigations would you do?

Blood investigations:
FBC, coagulation screen, U&Es/Cr, LFT, **GXM** (see Chapter • •)
Colorectal examination:
1. DRE (essential): r/o rectal tumours
2. Proctoscopy: anorectal pathology (haemorrhoids/fissure)
3. Rigid sigmoidoscopy: tumour/haemorrhoids
4. Flexible sigmoidoscopy: diverticular disease/left-sided tumours/colitis
5. Colonoscopy: visualises whole colon, and permits biopsy.
Imaging: double contrast barium enema, to r/o diverticular disease/ tumour/colitis.
Other: Stool culture to r/o infective cause.

What is the incidence of diverticular disease?

1/3 of the population in the Western world has **diverticulosis** (the incidental presence of colonic diverticulae) by age 60 years.

What causes a diverticular bleed?

Erosion into a bowel wall blood vessel by an adjacent diverticulum.

What is the treatment of a diverticular bleed?

The majority of diverticular bleeds will settle with **conservative management** (80–90%).
Resuscitate the patient with IV fluids, and place on bed rest. Consider transfusion if large volume of blood lost. Consider antibiotics if LIF pain/tenderness and/or raised WCC (diverticulitis.)

If not settling with conservative Mx, angiography and embolisation may be required, or resection of the affected bowel segment (10%).

What is angiodysplasia?

A common condition of the over 60s, usually affecting the right colon. Histologically it consists of thin-walled vascular channels in the submucosa. Patients present with massive PR bleeding or anaemia from slower chronic bleeding.
Rx: as with diverticular bleed.

CHAPTER 22: ABDOMINAL AORTIC ANEURYSM: LEAKAGE AND RUPTURE

APPLIED ANATOMY

What are the branches of the abdominal aorta from superior to inferior?	**Unpaired:** 1. Coeliac trunk 2. Superior mesenteric a. 3. Inferior mesenteric a. 4. Median sacral a. (at bifurcation). **Paired (visceral):** 1. Suprarenal (adrenal) aa. 2. Renal aa. 3. Gonadal aa. (ovarian/testicular). **Paired (abdominal wall):** 1. Subcostal aa. 2. Inferior phrenic aa. 3. Lumbar aa. (5 on each side). See figure 30.1, p. 264.
Where does the aorta span from?	T12 (behind median arcuate ligament) to L4.
What happens to it at L4?	Bifurcates into the left and right common iliac aa.
Where is the aorta in relation to the IVC?	The aorta lies slightly to the left of the IVC.
Which renal artery is longer?	The right renal a. due to the aorta being slightly displaced to the left.
What are the branches of the coeliac trunk?	1. Hepatic a. 2. Left gastric a. 3. Splenic a.
How does an AAA present?	1. Asymptomatic incidental finding on examination or on scanning for other reasons 2. Pulsatile, expansile mass in the abdomen (commonly the epigastrium) may cause epigastric or back pain (leaking aneurysm) 3. As an emergency ruptured aneurysm.

What are the features of ruptured AAA?

A triad of the following:
1. **Pain** in the epigastrium, radiating to the back
2. **Hypotension** with collapse and loss of consciousness
3. **Epigastric mass**: tender, pulsatile and expansile.

There *may* also be loss of peripheral pulses.

What is the difference between pulsatile and expansile?

A pulsatile mass may simply be transmitting a pulse from another structure eg enlarged para-aortic nodes. An expansile mass indicates an artery.

What is the management of ruptured AAA?

1. Oxygen via face mask
2. 2 large bore IV cannulae and IV fluids
3. Catheterise
4. Call for senior help; inform theatre and anaesthetist.

What investigations should be performed?

Blood investigations:
1. FBC: Hb level to assess blood loss
2. U+Es/Cr: assess renal function (?pre-renal failure 2ry to hypotension)
3. Amylase: r/o pancreatitis (epigastric pain)
4. GXM 6 units blood (*vital!*).

Imaging: Portable ultrasound is useful if available, or CT scan will confirm diagnosis, but *do not delay theatre by performing imaging in unstable patients*.

What is the principle of hypotensive resuscitation?

The judicial use of IV fluids to resuscitate the patient whilst keeping the systolic BP <100 mmHg. If BP rises, a formed clot may be blown off the rupture site and bleeding may be exacerbated.

What are the treatment options?

Endovascular repair, or open repair, using Dacron or PTFE graft.

What is the mortality rate of a ruptured AAA?

90% total; of the patients who make it to the OT, mortality is 50%.

What are the specific complications of AAA repair?

Early complications:
1. Ischaemic bowel (mesenteric a. usually involved in the aneurysm)
2. Renal failure (if aneurysm extends above renal aa.)
3. Leaking from anastomoses
4. Reperfusion injury (iliac aa. clamped during op are un-clamped; toxin build-up during clamping is released into general circulation)
5. Compartment syndrome of the lower limbs
6. 'Trash foot' (loosened atheromata embolise distally causing ischaemic phenomena).

Late complications:
1. Re-rupture
2. Erosion of the graft into GI tract (**aorto-enteric fistula**), causing massive haematemesis and death if no intervention made (this is ↓ by wrapping graft in the native aorta at time of repair)
3. Impotence.

CHAPTER 23: THE ACUTELY ISCHAEMIC LIMB AND AMPUTATION

THE ACUTELY ISCHAEMIC LIMB

How does a patient with acute limb ischaemia present?

With the 6 Ps.

What are the 6 Ps of acute limb ischaemia?

Pain
Pallor
Paraesthesia
Paralysis
Pulslessness
Perishingly cold (**p**oikilothermia).

What are the most likely causes of acute limb ischaemia?

Any sources of emboli:
Left side of heart:
- Atrial fibrillation (most common cause)
- MI (clot forming on dead muscle)
- Cardiomyopathy (clotted stagnant blood)
- Infective endocarditis (embolus of infected valvular vegetations)
- Atrial myxoma (rare).

Aneurysms (embolus of thrombotic material within the aneurysm: **thromboembolism**).
Atheromatous plaques (thromboembolism).
Right side of heart: **rare**; caused by venous clot (eg from DVT) entering arterial circulation via a patent atrial septal defect. Known as a **paradoxical embolus**.
Tumours.
Acute thrombosis:
Intra-arterial injection
Trauma
Popliteal aneurysm thrombosis.

What is distal lower limb ischaemia secondary to thromboembolism called?

Trash foot.

Where are emboli most likely to lodge?

At arterial bifurcations. Most common site of embolus lodging is in the superficial femoral artery at Hunter's canal.

How is embolism treated?

As a **surgical emergency**!

What is the first step?

Anticoagulate: start a heparin infusion.

Then what?

Determine whether occlusion is above knee (ie at superficial femoral a.) or below knee (can be determined clinically or with arteriogram):
If above knee: **embolectomy**
If below knee: **thrombolysis** (use streptokinase).

How is an embolectomy performed?

With a **Fogarty catheter**. This is a catheter with a balloon tip. Tip is passed distal to clot and balloon is inflated with saline. Catheter is then retracted, thus pulling the clot out. Embolectomy can be done under LA or GA.

How is acute thrombosis treated?

Also as a **surgical emergency**!

What first?

Anticoagulate: start heparin infusion.

Then what?

Get an **arteriogram** and determine **run-off**.

What is run-off and why is it important?

Run-off is an indication of how much blood is perfusing distal to the obstruction via **collateral circulation**:
Run-off present: **by-pass surgery**
Run-off absent: **thrombolysis +/– amputation**

What is the danger of successfully treating acute ischaemia?	Reperfusion injury.
What is this?	During the ischaemic period, toxins (eg lactate, myoglobin and K^+) build up. Reperfusion of the limb causes circulation of these toxins with risk of arrhythmias, ARDS and renal failure.
What is the other danger of reperfusion?	Compartment syndrome.
What is this?	It comprises the following events:

$\uparrow$ pressure in the fascial compartments of the limb secondary to oedema (in this case)

$\downarrow$

$\downarrow$ venous outflow

$\downarrow$

further $\uparrow$ in intra-compartmental pressure

$\downarrow$

compromised arterial inflow

$\downarrow$

muscle ischaemia and necrosis

What is the most important sign in compartment syndrome?	**Pain,** specifically: Pain out of proportion with the history Pain on passive stretching of affected muscles Pain on palpation of affected muscle groups.
What are the other signs?	The other 5 Ps. **Note:** Pulselessness, paraesthesia, pallor and perishingly cold are **late signs** in compartment syndrome!
What is the treatment for comfirmed compartment syndrome?	Fasciotomy: surgically cutting open fascia of all affected compartments.

Name some other causes besides reperfusion	Crush injury Fractures (open and closed) Tight plaster of Paris.

AMPUTATION

What are the indications for limb amputation?	*mnemonic:* **The 3 Ds** **D**ead limb (eg peripheral vascular disease causing critical ischaemia/ gangrene; most common reason in UK) **D**ead loss (eg trauma, neurological disease) **D**eadly (eg osteosarcoma, septic limb).
What type of lower limb amputations do you know of?	Above knee amputation (AKA) Below knee amputation (BKA) Symes amputation (at level of ankle joint) Transmetatarsal amputation Digit (ray) amputation.
What is the major difference between AKA and BKA besides the level?	The flaps: AKA: flaps are equal length BKA: long posterior flap (anterior flap less vascularised).
Is a tourniquet used in amputation?	Yes.
When would you *not* use one?	In peripheral vascular disease.
What are the complications of limb amputation?	Bleeding Breakdown of flaps (2ry to flap ischaemia) Flap retraction causing bone exposure Stump infection (esp. gas gangrene) +/− osteomyelitis Painful neuromas Ulceration Phantom limb pain

What is phantom limb pain? Pt. experiences pain in a limb which is no longer there (cerebral imprinting). Treat pharmacologically eg with tricyclic antidepressants or gabapentin.

CHAPTER 24: FURUNCLES, CARBUNCLES AND ABSCESSES

What is a furuncle?

An infection of a hair follicle resulting in a small collection of pus. Usually due to a **staphylococcal** infection. (Syn: **boil**).
Rx: none usually necessary; iodine may hasten resolution.

What is a carbuncle?

A collection of furuncles with subcutaneous connections and multiple drainage sites. Common in diabetes. Rx: as with furuncles, but consider penicillin, esp. in diabetics.

What is an abscess?

A collection of pus.

What is pus?

A thick fluid consisting of inflammatory exudates, live and dead polymorphs, and live and dead bacteria.

How does an abscess present?

With the classic signs of **inflammation**:
Rubor: redness
Calor: heat
Dolor: pain
Tumor: swelling
Functio laesa: loss of function
There may also be general symptoms of pyrexia (classically **swinging**) and rigors.

What is the treatment for an abscess?

Incision and drainage (I&D). Antibiotics will *not* cure an abscess as penetration into pus is **poor**.

How is I&D performed?

An incision (**cruciform** or **elliptical**) is made at the area of **pointing** (point of maximal fluctuance; represents point of least resistance for purulent discharge). Pus is evacuated and all **loculations** (pockets of pus) are broken down digitally or with help of a **curette**. Irrigation is performed with saline or betadine solution, and cavity is packed with kaltostat or ribbon gauze. This keeps the cavity open, allowing it to granulate from the bottom up (hence minimising recurrence).

What factors can predispose to abscess formation?

Immunodeficient states, such as diabetes, chemotherapy, and AIDS. **IVDU** (abscesses occur at injection sites).

What type of abscesses do you know of in general surgery?

1. Skin
2. Anorectal
3. Pilonidal
4. Breast
5. Intra-abdominal:
    a. Subphrenic
    b. Subhepatic
    c. Pelvic
    d. Pancreatic (see Chapter 17)
    e. Empyema of gallbladder (see Chapter 16)
    f. Renal
6. Intra-thoracic:
    a. Lung
    b. Pleural empyema
7. Tuberculous.

SKIN ABSCESS

Where do skin abscesses usually occur?

On the trunk and limbs. Also injection sites in IVDUs. Usually **staphylococcal**.
Rx: I&D (see above).

ANORECTAL ABSCESS

What do they arise from?

Infected anal glands within the anal canal.

See Figure 24.1:

The 1ry anal gland abscess (left of the diagram) may spread into the perianal region (**1 and 3**), or into the ischiorectal region (**2**), giving rise to the following (right of the diagram):

Submucous abscess (**A**) 5%

Perianal abscess (**B**) 60%

Ischiorectal abscess (**C**) 30%.

Pelvirectal abscesses (**D**) are essentially pelvic abscesses (they occur above levator ani) and arise from pelvic conditions such as appendicitis, PID, endometritis and **abdominal Crohn's disease**.

Figure 24.1 Anorectal abscess

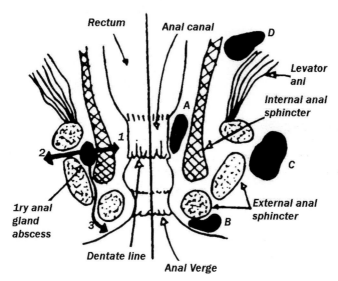

What is the treatment?	Depends on the type:
	Perianal: I&D
	Ischiorectal: I&D in the first instance. EUA once inflammation has settled: look for **fistulae-in-ano** which have an increased incidence in these abscesses (see Chapter 30b).
	Submucous: I&D under direct vision with proctoscope
	Pelvirectal: As with pelvic abscesses (see below).
What must an anorectal abscess be differentiated from?	A **buttock abscess**, which occurs on the skin of the buttock and is treated with simple I&D.
If in doubt, what can help in differentiating?	Pus culture: anorectal abscesses grow coliforms, while buttock abscesses mostly grow *Staphylococcus aureus*.

PILONIDAL ABSCESS

What is a pilonidal abscess?	An abscess arising from a **pilonidal sinus**.
What is a pilonidal sinus?	A short tract occurring at the **natal cleft** containing hairs. Postulated to be caused by implantation of hairs at the cleft due to prolonged sitting and friction. More common in **hirsute** (hairy) people. (Syn: **jeep bottom**, as soldiers frequently got them following long jeep rides!)
What is the treatment?	I&D. High risk of recurrence, so F/U needed for formal excision of sinus.

BREAST ABSCESS

| **Who are most prone to these?** | Breast-feeding mothers: bacteria enter cracks in the nipples caused by feeding. |

What is the most common organism found?	*Staphylococcus aureus.* (Also TB, syphilis and actinomycosis)
How is it treated?	Needle aspiration (use USS-guidance if within breast tissue) and flucloxacillin. I&D only if not responding to above and patient is becoming systemically unwell (drain breast of milk with breast pump first!)
Can a woman with a breast abscess breast-feed?	Yes, but from the unaffected breast only.
Can non-lactating women also develop breast abscesses?	Yes.
What must be ruled out?	Underlying carcinoma. Perform triple assessment (see Chapter 43).

INTRA-ABDOMINAL ABSCESS

What are the causes of intra-abdominal abscess?	1. Perforated viscus 2. Leakage during intra-abdominal surgery 3. Peritonitis.
What types do you know of?	**Subphrenic** (taken to mean 'true' subphrenic and subhepatic; see below) and **pelvic.** *(Note: pancreatic abscess, empyema of the gallbladder and renal abscess are also technically intra-abdominal abscesses but are usually discussed as separate entities. The former two can be found in their relevant chapters [17 and 16, respectively], whilst renal abscess is discussed separately below.)*
Where do subphrenic abscesses occur?	On the right side between the liver and the diaphragm (**'true' subphrenic**) and below the liver

(**subhepatic**). These can be further sub-divided into:
- L and R subphrenic (divided by **falciform ligament**)
- L and R subhepatic (lesser sac and pouch of Rutherford Morrison respectively).

Where do pelvic abscesses occur?

In the **pouch of Douglas** (between rectum and bladder in males, and rectum and vagina in females).

Can you give causes of each?

Subphrenic:
- Perforated peptic ulcer (localised collection)
- Gallbladder perforation
- Colonic perforation (eg 2ry to tumour).

Pelvic:
- Perforated inflamed appendix
- Perforated peptic ulcer (peptic secretions tracking down **right paracolic gutter**)
- Leaking distal bowel anastomosis
- Colorectal perforation (eg 2ry to tumour)
- Diverticular abscess
- Gynaecological pathology (eg PID, salpingitis).

How does an intra-abdominal abscess present?

Swinging fever, abdominal pain, nausea, vomiting, and malaise. Relevant history is important in elucidating cause, and will differ on suspected pathology (eg recent surgery, Hx of PUD, vaginal discharge).

What are the clinical findings?

General: unwell patient in pain
Hands: warm, tachycardia
Face: flushed, diaphoretic
Abdomen: peritonism; tender mass may be palpable in subphrenic abscess.

What are the investigations?	**Bloods:** FBC: ↑↑WBC U+Es: esp. if vomiting G&S: may need laparotomy. **Radiology:** **Erect CXR:** may show the following: – r/o air under diaphragm in perforated viscus – air–fluid level under right hemi-diaphragm in subphrenic abscess – tenting of right hemi-diaphragm. **USS:** very good for picking abscesses up. **CT scan:** can also be used, especially in pelvic abscesses.
What is the treatment?	1. Admit 2. NBM 3. IVF to correct electrolyte imbalances 4. IV antibiotics (broad spectrum, eg cef/gent/metro). This is **conservative**, and regular re-assessment of clinical status and radiology is important. If this fails, then: **Subphrenic:** – **Percutaneous drainage** under radiological guidance – Surgical drainage at laparotomy **Pelvic:** – **Digital drainage** via a rectal examination (put pressure over area of pointing) – Surgical drainage (percutaneous drainage not applicable).
What types of hepatic abscesses do you know?	Pyogenic (ie bacterial), amoebic, and hydatid.

What are their differences?   See Table 24.1.

Table 24.1

	Pyogenic	Amoebic	Hydatid
Causative organism(s)	• *E. coli* • *Klebsiella* • *Proteus* • *Bacteroides*	• *Entamoeba histolytica*	• *Echinococcus granulosus* • *Echinococcus multilocularis*
Mode of spread	Intra-abdominal pathology: cholangitis, diverticulitis, liver cancer/ mets	Faeco-oral transmission	Zoonosis: exposure to dogs, sheep, cattle (all carriers)
Presentation	**Fever** **Chills** **RUQ pain** Jaundice Weight loss	**Fever** **RUQ pain** Chills (much less) Diarrhoea Jaundice	RUQ pain Jaundice
	Signs: hepatomegaly, RUQ tenderness, jaundice		
Investigations	**Blood investigations** FBC: ↑WCC LFT: all raised	**Blood investigations** FBC: ↑WCC LFT: all raised	**Blood investigations** FBC: ↑WCC LFT: all raised
	Imaging: USS/CTscan (AXR may show calcified cyst with hydatid disease)		
		Special tests Serological test for *Entamoeba* antibodies (↑ 95%)	**Special tests** 1. Serological test for *Echinococcus* antibodies 2. **Casoni skin test**

Table 24.1 (continued)

	Pyogenic	**Amoebic**	**Hydatid**
Treatment	1. Abx: cef/ gent/met 2. Percutaneous image guided drainage 3. Surgical drainage if above has failed	1. Abx: metro 2. Surgical drainage if not responsive to Abx	1. Anti-parasitic: mebendazole, followed by surgical excision of cyst (*no aspiration as risk of anaphylaxis to organism!*)

What are the major risks with hydatid cysts?

Erosion into pleural cavity, pericardial sac or biliary tree; or **rupture** into peritoneal cavity causing **anaphylactic shock**.

What types of renal abscesses do you know of?

Pyonephrosis and **perinephric abscess**.

How do they mainly differ from subphrenic and pelvic abscesses?

They are **retroperitoneal** as opposed to **intraperitoneal**.

How do they differ from each other?

Pyonephrosis occurs when the PUJ becomes obstructed during a **pyelonephritis**. This results in back-up of pus into a **hydronephrotic** kidney (the kidney literally becomes a bag of pus). **Rx:** percutaneous or surgical drainage followed by **pyeloplasty** (surgical correction of the hydronephrosis).
Perinephric abscess occurs when pyelonephritis occurs in a kidney containing a **staghorn calculus** (large calculus forming a cast of all the renal calyces). Pus cannot drain and discharges through the renal capsule into the perinephric space.

The resulting abscess may point towards the **flank**.
Rx: I&D followed later by **nephrectomy**.

What organisms are present? Mostly *E. coli* and *Proteus*.

INTRATHORACIC ABSCESS

What types do you know of? **Lung abscess** and **lung empyema** (syn. **empyema thoracis**).

What causes lung abscess? Two main causes:
- Bacterial pneumonia
- Aspiration of gastric contents (**Mendelson's syndrome**); usually a **sterile** abscess.

How does it present? Swinging pyrexia, foul smelling sputum, haemoptysis, and malaise.

What is the investigation of choice? Erect CXR: shows a cavitating shadow +/− air–fluid level.

Which bacteria are usually responsible in pneumonia? *Stophylococcus aureus*, *Streptococcus pneumonia*, *Pseudomonas*, *Klebsiella.*

What is the treatment? Antibiotics; percutaneous drainage if this fails.

What is lung empyema? Pus in the pleural space usually caused by superinfection of a pleural effusion.

How does it present? Also with a swinging pyrexia, but respiratory distress may be apparent.

What does the CXR show? Blunting of the costo-diaphragmatic (C-D) angles.

What is the treatment? Depends on the stage (3 stages in all):
Exudative phase: pus is free-flowing; can be adequately treated by chest tube drainage and antibiotics.
Fibrinopurulent phase: often associated with the development of

thick pus and multiple loculations. Simple drainage and antibiotics inadequate. Surgical intervention to evacuate infected material and create a unified space for drainage. **Organisation stage:** fibrotic encasement of the lung requiring more complex surgical procedures for infection control and eradication, such as **decortication** and suction drainage usually resulting in lung re-expansion.

TUBERCULOUS ABSCESS

What is a tuberculous abscess?

An abscess caused by *Mycobacterium tuberculosis*. (Syn: **cold abscess**).

How might one present?

As a swelling anywhere in the body, but unlike other abscesses, pain and redness are usually **absent** (hence its synonymous name above).

Where do they classically present?

In the neck due to suppuration of cervical lymph nodes.

What is the treatment?

I&D and anti-tuberculous drug therapy.

What is the risk?

Formation of a draining sinus.

How else might a cold abscess present?

As a **psoas abscess**.

How does this arise?

From pre-existing tuberculous infection of the vertebral bodies (**Pott's disease**). Pus tracks from the vertebrae (usually T12–L1 ie the insertion of psoas major) to the psoas major.

What are the clinical features?

Generally, there will be signs and symptoms of tuberculosis (weight loss, night sweats, persistent non-productive cough).

On examination, there may be a **mass in the RIF**. If presenting late, pus may track down further along the length of psoas major and present as an abscess in the **groin**. In *very late* presentations, the pus may leave psoas to track further down and present as a **medial thigh** abscess at **Hunter's canal** via the **femoral triangle**.

What is Hunter's canal?

Boundaries: gutter-shaped groove between vastus medialis and the adductor muscles that is roofed by fascia.
Contents: femoral a. & v., saphenous n. and n. to vastus medialis.
(Syn. **adductor** or **subsartorial canal.**)

What is the femoral triangle?

Boundaries: inguinal ligament, medial border of sartorius and *medial* border of adductor longus. It abuts Hunter's canal from above.
Floor: iliasus, **psoas**, pectineus and adductor longus.
Contents: femoral vessels and nerve.

Can a psoas abscess be picked up

Yes, there will be loss of the psoas shadow on **AXR** on the affected side. USS or CT scan, however, are the imaging studies of choice.

Is a psoas abscess *always* cold?

No, it can less commonly be pyogenic (hot), and is usually due to a **paracolic abscess** (abscess lying in the paracolic gutter, caused by any of the causes of subphrenic or pelvic abscesses; see above).

CHAPTER 25: BURNS

What types of burns do you know of?
Thermal, electrical, chemical and friction burns.

How are burns classified?
As **partial thickness** and **full thickness**. Partial thickness is further subdivided into **epidermal** and **superficial dermal** burns.

How do they differ clinically?
Epidermal: Patient complains of **pain.**
Inspection: erythematous, involving only the epidermis.
Palpation: exquisitely **tender**.
(Syn: **1st degree burns**; eg sunburn, flash burns.)
Superficial dermal: Patient complains of **pain**.
Inspection: erythematous with **blistering** and possible epidermal loss.
Palpation: exquisitely **tender**. (Syn. **2nd degree burns**.)
Full thickness: Pain is variable.
Inspection: dull grey/white. Presence of **eschar** (see below).
Palpation: Usually **insensate** to touch with a **leathery** feel.
(Syn. **3rd degree burns**.)

What is the rule of 9s?
Clinical measure of the % of total body surface area (TBSA) involved in a burn (see Figure 25.1):
Upper limbs: 9% each (entire limb)
Lower limbs: 18% each (entire limb)
Trunk: 18% front, 18% back
Head: 9% (entire head)
Perineum & genitalia: 1% (total area).
For irregular burns, the patient's **palm size** can be estimated as 1% of TBSA and used to measure the area involved.

Figure 25.1 The Rule of 9s

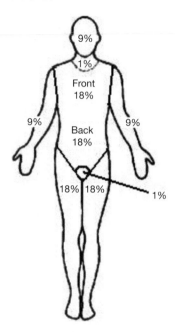

9%

1%

Front 18%

9% Back 18% 9%

18% 18% 1%

What is the immediate management?

Resuscitation! ABCs are paramount (see Chapter 11).
Airway: look for evidence of smoke inhalation (soot at nostrils/mouth; burnt nasal hairs; singed eyebrows) and **mucosal oedema** which may cause rapid airway obstruction (have a low threshold for intubation!)
Breathing: give O_2, especially if there was risk of smoke inhalation.
Circulation: fluids are especially important in burns patients as they lose fluids rapidly from burn site.
Disability: neurological status; if GCS altered, think smoke inhalation.
Exposure: Assess from head to toe for areas of burns and determine

TBSA. **Keep warm** as thermoregulation is compromised with ↑ burn area.
Then *and only then* can further management be instituted.

How much fluid would you give as an initial resuscitation?

According to the **Parkland formula:** 3–4 ml/kg body weight/% TBSA in first 24 h This calculated volume is given as: 1/2 in first 8 hours, then 1/2 in next 16 hours.

So how are the individual types treated?

Epidermal: basic wound care (keep clean, give analgesia, moisturise with cream).
Superficial dermal: aspirate blister fluid, but leave them intact (act as natural dressing); apply absorbent dressing (eg plastic films or hydrocolloids). Surgical intervention only if no healing by 2–3 weeks.
Full thickness: all need surgical intervention involving excision of burnt area (**eschar**) and application of a skin graft (or flap if necessary).

When is surgery particularly indicated?

In **circumferential full-thickness burns**. If involving the trunk, eschar may cause **respiratory distress** by physically restricting respiration. If involving limbs, eschar may cause **compartment syndrome**. An **escharotomy** is indicated (longitudinal incisions within eschar to release constriction).

What about antibiotics?

Controversial! All burns *will* become colonised with bacteria (usually *Staphylococcus aureus*). Regular swabs should be taken, and burnt areas should be checked regularly for evidence of **cellulitis**. If present, then antibiotics *should* be given (topical and/or oral). Otherwise, routine administration differs from centre to centre (check local policy).

What is the danger with electrical burns?

Cardiac arrhythmias and cardiac arrest (current usually passes through body to the earth). Perform an ECG.

How are chemical burns managed?

As above, but with copious initial irrigation and/or neutralisation (if applicable) especially if involving the eyes.

Which are more damaging: acids or alkalis?

Alkalis (body cannot buffer them, so longer effect).

CHAPTER 26: HAEMATURIA

What is haematuria?

The presence of blood in the urine. It may be microscopic or macroscopic (visible to the naked eye).

What are the causes?

Approach this anatomically:
General:
Bleeding dyscrasias
Anticoagulation therapy (warfarin, aspirin)
Liver disease (clotting impairment).
Kidney:
Calculi
Infection (**pyelonephritis** incl. TB)
Trauma
Carcinoma
Infarction (thromboembolic or sickle cell disease).
Ureter:
Calculi
Neoplasm.
Bladder:
Calculi
Infection (**cystitis** incl. TB; also schistosomiasis [**syn.** bilharzia])
Carcinoma.
Prostate:
Benign prostatic hyperplasia (BPH)
Prostatic carcinoma.
Urethra:
Calculi
Trauma (incl. rupture and traumatic catheterisation)
Infection (**urethritis**)
Carcinoma.

What is the most important clinical feature in distinguishing the cause of haematuria?

Associated pain. The following types of associated pain are matched with their most likely diagnoses:
No pain: urinary tract neoplasm (see Chapters 44 to 47)

Dull to sharp lumbar pain:
pyelonephritis, renal calculi or trauma
Colicky loin to groin pain: ureteric calculi
Suprapubic pain: cystitis or calculi
Dysuria: urethritis, calculi or trauma.

What other points in the history are important?

1. Past history or risk factors for calculi (see Chapter 34b)
2. Past history or risk factors for neoplasm (see Chapters 44 to 47)
3. Bleeding disorders, liver disease or anticoagulation therapy
4. Prior episodes of haematuria (eg past UTIs)
5. Recent travel or fresh water swimming (schistosomiasis)
6. Symptoms of anaemia.

How can the important points be remembered when assessing haematuria?

mnemonic: **SITTT**
Stones
Infection
Trauma
Tumour
Tuberculosis.

What are the significant findings on examination?

There may be symptoms of anaemia. A mass may be felt on balloting the kidneys. A **digital rectal examination** is *mandatory* to r/o prostate disease.

How is haematuria managed?

Urine dipstick: for leucocytes and nitrites (presence of *E. coli*), and to confirm microscopic haematuria
MSU: for microscopy, culture and sensitivity (?infection) and for cytology (?neoplasm)
Blood investigations:
1. FBC: ↓Hb if anaemic; ↑WBC if infection present (mostly in pyelonephritis)

2. BUN/Cr: assess renal function which may be deranged in renal disease or if there is an element of urinary retention (eg ureteric stone)
3. Clotting screen: PT/PTT and LFTs
4. G&S: if transfusion is needed
5. Urate: ?gout as a cause of calculi.

Imaging:
1. KUB: 90% of renal calculi are radio-opaque.
2. IVU: to assess position of calculi (if present) and degree of ureteric obstruction (if any); also outlines urinary tract neoplasms.
3. USS: also picks up stones but good for tumours as well.

Other: flexible cystoscopy (done under LA as a day case).

These tests all constitute a **haematuria screen**. The cause of haematuria is then treated appropriately (see relevant chapters).

What if there are clots in the urine?

Admit the pt. for catheterisation with a 3-way catheter and bladder irrigation as there is a risk of urinary retention.

CHAPTER 27: ACUTE TESTICULAR DISORDERS: TORSION AND EPIDIDYMO-ORCHITIS

TESTICULAR TORSION

What is torsion?	The twisting of the testicle on its vascular pedicle with resultant arterial occlusion and testicular infarction.
Who gets it?	Young men.
What is the classic history?	Acute onset of scrotal pain referred to the abdomen following vigorous physical activity (incl. sex) or minor trauma.
Why is pain referred to the abdomen?	The testes were abdominal structures before their descent. Visceral pain is therefore referred there.
What predisposes to torsion?	Abnormal attachment of tunica vaginalis to the testis: **Normal:** tunica vaginalis surrounds the anterior and lateral aspects of the body of the testis, and is attached to the posterior aspect of the testis and part of the epididymis, preventing twisting.

Figure 27.1 Testicular torsion

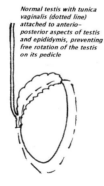

Normal testis with tunica vaginalis (dotted line) attached to anterio–posterior aspects of testis and epididymis, preventing free rotation of the testis on its pedicle

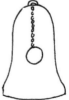

'Clapper–in–a–bell' deformity in which tunica vaginalis completely surrounds the testis and epididymis, allowing free rotation of the testis (clapper) around its pedicle within the tunica (bell)

Abnormal: tunica vaginalis surrounds the entire testis and epididymis, allowing twisting. This is the classic **bell clapper deformity**.

What is found clinically?

Swollen, tender, **high riding** testis with a **lateral** lie (**as opposed to the normal longitudinal lie**).

NB the other testis *must* be examined as the anatomical defect is frequently bilateral making torsion there equally as likely.

What is the number one differential?

Acute epididymo-orchitis.

Are there any investigations that can be used to aid in the diagnosis?

The diagnosis of torsion is a clinical one. However, if there is doubt, a **Doppler USS** can be performed to assess testicular blood flow. This, however, has low sensitivity and specificity. *When in doubt, treat as torsion!*

What is the treatment?

Emergent surgical exploration with untorting of the testis. Once untorted, wrap in warm towels to encourage blood flow:
If viable: invaginate (sew back) tunica vaginalis and fix testis to scrotum (**orchidopexy**).
If not viable: remove testis (**orchidectomy**).

Should the unaffected testis be explored as well?

Yes! An orchidopexy should be performed on this one too.

How long is the window of opportunity for release of torsion from time of onset?

6 hours, after which time the risk of testicular infarction greatly increases.

ACUTE EPIDIDYMO-ORCHITIS

What is it?
Acute infection of the epididymis and testis.

Who gets it?
Males of all ages.

What are the organisms?
Young and old: *E. coli*
Young adults: STDs such as gonorrhoea and chlamydia
Mumps may also affect the testes causing a viral orchitis (usually bilateral).

What is the history?
Insidious or acute onset of painful, tender testis. History may be very similar to torsion.

What is found clinically?
Swollen, tender testis and/or epididymis with an erythematous scrotum. Testis is not generally high riding.

What is the number one differential?
Acute testicular torsion.

How can the two be distinguished?
May be impossible clinically, but the time interval may give a clue: acute epididymo-orchitis may begin insidiously and worsen gradually over days. After only 6 hours, a torted testis may become infracted and the patient can become gravely ill and possibly septic.

What is the treatment?
Anti-inflammatory medications and antibiotics for 4–6 weeks.

B. Non-acute General Surgical conditions

CHAPTER 28: ABDOMINAL WALL: HERNIAE

What is a hernia?

A protrusion of a viscus through an abnormal opening or weakness in the wall of its containing cavity.

What types of abdominal wall herniae do you know of?

Inguinal (most common)
Femoral
Umbilical
Paraumbilical
Incisional
Epigastric.
Rare:
Spigelian
Lumbar
Obturator
Gluteal.
NB hiatus hernia is *not* an abdominal wall hernia, but a stomach herniation through the hiatal orifice of the diaphragm.

What factors predispose to abdominal wall herniation?

Any cause of ↑ intra-abdominal pressure, including:
Obesity
COPD
Pregnancy
Chronic cough
Constipation (forcing stool)
Urinary retention (forced micturition)
Ascites.
Also: Wound factors (incisional herniae; see below)
Appendicectomy (direct herniae; see below).

INGUINAL HERNIAE

APPLIED ANATOMY

Where does the inguinal ligament (of Poupart) run?

From the anterior superior iliac spine (ASIS) to to the pubic tubercle (approximately 1.5 cm lateral to the symphysis pubis).

What is the mid-inguinal point?

The midpoint of an imaginary line joining the ASIS to the symphysis pubis. This differs from the **mid-point of the inguinal ligament** which is slightly **lateral** (1 finger-breadth) to the mid-inguinal point.

What is the relevance of these two points?

2 cm below the **mid-inguinal point** is the anatomical landmark of:
- The femoral artery
- The femoral head.

The **mid-point of the inguinal ligament** is the anatomical landmark of the **internal** (or **deep**) **ring** of the inguinal canal.

What is the clinical significance of the pubic tubercle?

It is the anatomical landmark of the **external** (or **superficial**) **ring**.

What is the significance of the deep and superficial rings?

They are the entry and exit points respectively of the inguinal canal. The testis entered the canal via the deep ring, and entered the scrotum via the superficial ring during its descent, dragging the spermatic cord behind it. It, in turn, was dragged by the **gubernaculum**, which attaches it to the scrotum.

What are the boundaries of the inguinal canal?

Anterior wall formed by the external oblique aponeurosis, assisted laterally by the internal oblique muscle.

Posterior wall by the conjoint tendon medially and the transversalis fascia throughout.

Roof by the lower edge of internal oblique and transversus muscles, which medially join together as the **conjoint tendon** and insert onto the pubic crest and the pectineal line of pubic bone.

Floor by the in-rolled lower edge of the inguinal ligament, reinforced medially by the lacunar ligament.

What lies within the inguinal canal?

Males: spermatic cord
Females: round ligament.

What are the contents of the spermatic cord?

3 arteries:
1. testicular a. (from aorta)
2. a. to ductus (vas) deferens (from sup. vesical a.)
3. cremasteric a. (from inf. epigastric a.)

3 nerves:
1. genital branch of genitofemoral n.
2. ilioinguinal n. (lies *on* the cord)
3. sympathetic nn.

4 others:
1. pampiniform plexus (testicular venous drainage)
2. ductus (vas) deferens
3. lymphatics
4. processus vaginalis (when bowel pushes into this, it becomes the **hernial sac**).

What are the coverings of the spermatic cord?

3 in all, each derived during testicular descent. From inside out:
1. **Internal spermatic fascia:** derived from the transversalis fascia at the deep inguinal ring.
2. **Cremasteric fascia and muscle:** derived from the internal oblique and transversus fascia and muscles.

3. **External spermatic fascia:** derived from the external oblique aponeurosis.

CLINICAL CONSIDERATIONS

What are the differentials of an inguinal swelling?

When answering this, start superficially and go deep:
Skin and subcutaneous tissue:
- Lipoma

Within inguinal canal:
- Lipoma of the cord
- Undescended testis
- Vaginal hydrocele (ie one continuous with the peritoneum)

Nearby:
- Femoral hernia.

What types of inguinal herniae do you know of?

Direct and indirect.

What does an inguinal hernia usually contain?

Small bowel.

Should a hernia be examined with the patient standing or supine?

Both! If the pt. is standing, start examining in the standing position, and likewise for the supine position.

What should be commented on during examination of a hernia?

Inspection: obvious groin bulge, scrotal extension, scars (from previous hernia repair), skin changes, ?contralateral hernia present.
Palpation: tenderness, temperature, reducibility (let pt. do this!), control (see Table 28.1), expansile cough impulse, differentiation from other scrotal masses if scrotal extension is present (can you palpate spermatic cord above it? If yes, then unlikely to be a hernia). Palpate other side.
Auscultation: bowel sounds.

What are the differences between direct and indirect herniae?
See Table 28.1.

Table 28.1

	Indirect hernia	**Direct hernia**
Cause	Weakness at the deep ring	Weakness of the medial aspect of posterior wall (conjoint tendon)
Clinical anatomy	Bowel enters inguinal canal via deep ring and traverses the canal within a patent processus vaginalis (hernial sac)	Bowel does not enter canal, but causes a bulge in medial aspect of posterior wall behind the superficial ring
Scrotal extension	Possible if bowel exits the canal via superficial ring and descends into the scrotum (**inguinoscrotal hernia**)	Not possible as bowel does not enter canal (except *rarely* in extremely large herniae)
Control	Can be controlled after **reduction of herniated bowel** by digital pressure over the deep ring (1 finger-breadth lateral to the mid-inguinal point ie the mid-point of the inguinal ligament; see above)	Not controlled after reduction by digital pressure over the deep ring
Surgical anatomy	Hernia is *lateral* to **inferior epigastric artery** (which comes off the femoral a. and marks the mid-inguinal point at operation)	Hernia is *medial* to **inferior epigastric artery** and is seen bulging within **Hasselbach's triangle** (formed by conjoint tendon medially, inferior epigastric a. laterally and inguinal ligament inferiorly)

What is the best way to differentiate between a direct and indirect hernia?	At surgery!
Which operation predisposes to direct inguinal hernia?	Appendicectomy: ilioinguinal n. may be cut during incision. This nerve supplies the conjoint tendon which then becomes weak, leading to direct herniation.
What is an incarcerated hernia?	An irreducible, non-obstructed hernia. Caused by adhesions forming around the sac.
What are the risks of a hernia becoming incarcerated?	**Mechanical obstruction** (usually **small bowel** obstruction as this is the type of bowel which is most likely to herniate) and **strangulation**.
What is the precipitating factor?	A constricting hernial neck (eg the **deep ring** in indirect inguinal herniae).
What is a strangulated hernia?	A hernia containing ischaemic bowel (see Mechanical Obstruction under Chapter 18). Obstruction usually precedes strangulation (except in Richter's hernia; see below).
What are the clinical features of a strangulated hernia?	A tense, tender, irreducible hernia with absent bowel sounds.
What is reduction *en masse*?	Reduction of the **entire hernial sac** *including* the strangulated bowel and constricting neck. There is an ↑ risk of intra-abdominal perforation and generalised peritonitis.
What are the treatment options for inguinal herniae?	**Conservative:** a truss (special belt which applies pressure over inguinal defect, hence controlling hernia); unsatisfactory, and reserved for elderly patients who are unfit for anaesthesia.

Surgical: herniorrhaphy. Done electively in uncomplicated cases and emergently in cases of obstruction and strangulation. Types available:

- Laparoscopic herniorrhaphy
- Open herniorrhaphy:
  - Lichtenstein (mesh) repair: bowel reduced, deep ring tightened and **prolene mesh** applied to reinforce lax posterior wall (most common)
  - Shouldice repair: as above, but posterior wall is split and edges overlapped and tightened with prolene sutures.

Obstructed and strangulated bowel are dealt with accordingly (see Chapter 18).

What variants of inguinal herniae do you know of?

Pantaloon: both direct and indirect hernia occurring simultaneously, and resembling the legs of a pair of trousers straddling the inferior epigastric a. at operation (hence the name).

Richter's: a **knuckle** of bowel (from the **anti-mesenteric** border) becomes constricted in the neck of the hernial sac without causing complete intestinal lumen occlusion. More frequently found in femoral and obturator hernias. (**Syn.** levator hernia, partial enterocele or nipped hernia.)

Maydl's: a double loop hernia in which segments of bowel both proximal and distal to the central in-folded loop become incarcerated. The central loop is most prone to strangulation. (**Syn.** hernia-en-W because of shape.)

Sliding: part of hernial sac is formed by a viscus (eg caecum or bladder).
Littré's: hernial sac containing a Meckel's diverticulum.
Amyand's: hernial sac containing an inflamed appendix.

FEMORAL HERNIAE

APPLIED ANATOMY

Where does femoral herniation occur?	At the femoral canal.
What are the boundaries and contents of the femoral canal?	**Anterior:** the inguinal ligament **Posterior:** the pectineal (Cooper's) ligament **Medial:** the lacunar (Gimbernat's) ligament and iliopubic tract **Lateral:** the femoral vein **Contents:** fatty connective tissue and the deep inguinal node of Cloquet (drains lymph from the penis/clitoris).

CLINICAL CONSIDERATIONS

Are femoral herniae more common in males or females?	Females. F:M = 2.5:1.
Are femoral herniae the most common herniae in females then?	No! Inguinal herniae are still the most common.
Why are they more common in females?	The inguinal ligament makes a wider angle with the pubis. Pregnancy also $\uparrow$ intra-abdominal pressure.
What are the differentials of a femoral hernia?	Again, start superficially and work deep: *Skin and subcutaneous tissue:* • Lipoma.

Within the femoral canal:
- Saphena varix (saphenous v. varicosity)
- Enlarged node (of Cloquet)
- Ectopic testis.

Nearby:
- Inguinal hernia
- Femoral a. aneurysm
- Psoas abscess or bursa (posterior to canal).

What does a femoral hernia usually contain?

Omentum.

If it contains bowel, what type of bowel is it?

Small bowel, usually forming a Richter's hernia (see above).

How can a femoral hernia be distinguished clinically from an inguinal hernia?

By finding the **pubic tubercle**: A femoral hernia occurs **below and lateral** to the pubic tubercle. An inguinal hernia occurs **above and medial** to it.

How should a femoral hernia be treated?

Urgently. There is a high risk of ischaemia of the contents as 3 sides of the canal (anterior, posterior and medial) are relatively rigid structures, not allowing for expansion.

What are the treatment options?

All surgical:
Abdominal/extraperitoneal/ suprapubic approach: is used when obstruction or strangulation is suspected or present; in patients who have undergone previous groin surgery; and in bilateral cases where both sides can be repaired simultaneously.
Inguinal/high operation: is best used when there is a concomitant primary inguinal hernia on the same side that can be repaired simultaneously.

Crural/low operation: is recommended for the easily reducible uncomplicated femoral hernia especially in the thin patient when it can be undertaken electively using local anaesthesia.

OTHER TYPES OF HERNIAE

What is the difference between an umbilical and paraumbilical hernia?

An **umbilical hernia** occurs through a weakness in the actual umbilical cicatrix (scar).
A **paraumbilical hernia** occurs through a defect *adjacent* to the cicatrix.

Who are more prone to getting these herniae?

Afro-Caribbean populations.

What is the usual content?

Both usually contain omentum.

What are the treatment options?

Surgical. Either a **mesh repair** or a **Mayo repair** is done. In both, the hernia is reduced and the sac is excised. Then, in the former, a prolene mesh is used to close the defect. In the latter, the cut edges are overlapped ('vest over pants') and sutured together with prolene.

What is the rule of 3s in umbilical herniae in infants?

1. Occurs in **3%** of live births
2. Only **3:1000** need repair
3. Repair done only after **age 3**
4. Recur in **3rd trimester** of pregnancy.

How does an epigastric hernia usually present?

As an epigastric swelling which may cause discomfort and is occasionally painful.

What is the main differential?

A lipoma.

What does it usually contain?

Omentum.

How is it treated?	As with umbilical and paraumbilical herniae.
What are the predisposing factors for incisional herniae?	Anything affecting proper wound healing: **General:** Age Immunosuppression Obesity Malnutrition **Wound:** Poor wound closure technique Infection (incl. nearby stoma) Haematoma Foreign body (incl. drains) **Incision type:** Longitudinal incisions.
Which incision has the lowest incidence of incisional hernia?	Pfannensteil incisions.
What is a Spigelian hernia?	One which herniates through the **linea semilunaris**. *Rare.*
What is the linea semilunaris?	The lateral edge of the fascia enclosing rectus abdominis.
What is an obturator hernia?	One which herniates through the obturator canal of the pelvis. Occurs in F>M, and is most commonly of the Richter's variety.
What is a lumbar hernia?	One which herniates through the posteriorly situated lumbar triangle (of Petit). Its boundaries are: iliac crest, posterior external oblique and anterior latissimus dorsi.
What is a gluteal hernia?	One which herniates through the greater sciatic notch of the pelvis.

CHAPTER 29: UPPER GASTROINTESTINAL TRACT DISORDERS

a. OESOPHAGUS

APPLIED ANATOMY

What is the oesophagus?	A muscular tube extending from the cricoid cartilage (C6) to the gastro-oesophageal junction (T10).
What is the distance from the top incisor teeth to the gastro-oesophageal junction?	40 cm.
How long is the oesophagus?	25 cm.
What is it lined with?	Stratified squamous epithelium.
What type of muscle is it made of?	Depends on the level: Upper 1/3: striated Middle 1/3: striated and smooth Lower 1/3: smooth The muscles themselves are arranged as an outer longitudinal layer and an inner circular layer.
What are its narrowest points?	There are 3 (distances given are measured from the front incisor teeth): 1. Cricopharyngeal sphincter (15 cm) 2. At the aortic arch (22 cm) 3. Where it crosses the diaphragm (38 cm).
How much of the oesophagus is intra-abdominal?	2 cm.

What are the phases of swallowing?	Oral → Pharyngeal → Oesophageal.
What is difficulty in swallowing called?	Dysphagia.
What are the causes?	**Intraluminal causes:** Foreign body Oesophageal webs. **Mural (oesophageal wall) causes:** Benign strictures (secondary to chronic acid reflux) Oesophageal tumours (benign or malignant). **Extraluminal causes:** Oesophageal diverticulum Pharyngeal pouch Lymphadenopathy Goitre Aortic aneurysm Paraoesophageal (rolling) hiatus hernia.
What is *painful* swallowing called?	Odynophagia.
What motility disorders do you know of?	Achalasia Chagas' disease Pharyngeal pouch Diffuse oesophageal spasm (DOS).
How do they present?	See Table 29.1.
What other conditions are associated with Chagas' disease?	Cardiomyopathy, megaduodenum, megacolon and megaureter.

Table 29.1

	Achalasia	Chagas' disease	Pharyngeal pouch	DOS
Epidemiology	M=F; age: 30–60 Worldwide	M=F; all ages Endemic in Brazil	M>F; elderly Worldwide	M>F; middle-aged Worldwide
Definition	Failure of LOS to relax	Failure of LOS to relax	Pulsion diverticulum of the pharynx through gap in inferior constrictor (**Killian's** dehiscence)	Spasms of the oesophagus causing anginal type pain
Cause	Unknown	Chronic infection with *Trypanosoma cruzi* causing destruction of intermuscular ganglion cells	Uncoordinated swallowing	Unknown
Presents	Dysphagia for solids and liquids **in equal amounts**	Dysphagia for solids and liquids **in equal amounts**	Halitosis, early regurgitation of food, sore throat, dysphagia and neck swelling	Angina-type pain
Barium swallow	**Bird beak** appearance; dilated oesophagus; no gastric bubble	**Bird beak** appearance; dilated oesophagus; no gastric bubble	Pouch is visualised	**Corkscrew** appearance
Manometry	↑ pressure; no peristalsis	↑ pressure; no peristalsis	N/A	**Nutcracker** oesophagus
Treatment	Balloon dilation or **Heller's cardiomyotomy**	Balloon dilation or **Heller's cardiomyotomy**	Open or laparoscopic (**Dohlman's**) excision	Nifedipine and balloon dilation

What is GORD?	Reflux of acidic stomach contents (gastric juice) into the distal oesophagus causing mucosal irritation.
What usually prevents this reflux?	Lower oesophageal sphincter (LOS).
Is this a true anatomical sphincter?	No. It is more of a physiological one, thought to act by a combination of factors:

    1. The angle at which the oesophagus enters the stomach cardia (cardio-oesophageal angle).
    2. The pinch-cock effect of the diaphragm as the oesophagus passes through its hiatus.
    3. Transmitted intra-abdominal pressure compressing distal oesophagus.

What is the cause of GORD?	Thought to be an alteration of the above LOS dynamics. **Hiatus hernia** (see under *Stomach* below) *may* contribute, but not everyone with hiatus hernia has GORD and vice-versa. Other contributing factors include alcohol (relaxing effect on sphincter), ↑ intra-abdominal pressure (as in pregnancy), obesity, prolonged immobilisation and gastric CA.
What are the symptoms?	Retrosternal burning sensation that rises up the chest (**heartburn**; most common, may mimic angina) Dyspepsia Nocturnal cough (acid seeps up oesophagus while patient is asleep in the supine position and irritates pharyngeal mucosa)

Post-nasal drip (thought to be caused by hypersensitivity of irritated pharyngeal mucosa to normal post-nasal secretions which, in the normal patient, usually occurs unnoticed).

NB It is postulated that many ENT ailments such as otitis media and Eustachian tube dysfunction may be because of a direct effect of GORD.

What is found on examination?

Very little. There may be signs of **poor dentition** due to acidic tooth erosion from nocturnal rising acid while supine.

What is the major risk of GORD?

Barrett's oesophagus.

What is Barrett's oesophagus?

Metaplastic change of the distal oesophageal mucosa 2ry to prolonged acidic irritation. The normal squamous epithelium changes to columnar epithelium, resembling gastric mucosa. The **gastro-oesophageal junction** *rises*. This is a **pre-malignant** condition.

What is the risk of developing carcinoma from a Barrett's oesophagus?

It is increased 40-fold.

What type of carcinoma is it?

Adenocarcinoma (see Chapter 36).

What are the investigations for GORD?

Imaging: barium meal; shows reflux +/– hiatus hernia.
Other: oesophagogastroduodenoscopy (**OGD**); the following can be achieved:
- Direct visualisation of reflux and Barrett's Oesophagus (seen as **'tongues'** of gastric mucosa crawling upwards; can be graded)
- pH studies to confirm diagnosis

- Biopsies in suspected cases of Barrett's oesophagus.

What is the management?

Conservative: simple measures first:
- Stop smoking and alcohol
- Lose weight
- No tight clothing (eg corsets)
- Small, regular meals instead of large ones
- Avoid sleeping immediately after meals
- Raise head of bed at night (mechanical avoidance of reflux)
- $\downarrow$ acid secretion:
  - Antacid preparations
  - H_2-antagonists (eg ranitidine)
  - Proton pump inhibitors (PPIs; eg omeprazole).

Most cases resolve with these measures.

Surgical: performed in severe cases resistant to conservative measures:

Nissen's fundoplication is the treatment of choice. The fundus of stomach is wrapped around the gastro-oesophageal junction, and acts as a sphincter during gastric motility, preventing reflux.

b. STOMACH

APPLIED ANATOMY

Name the parts of the stomach.

See Figure 29.1.

What is the origin of the stomach's blood supply?

The coeliac trunk, a branch of the abdominal aorta.

What comprises the stomach bed?

Upper part of left kidney
Pancreas
Spleen
Left suprarenal (adrenal) gland

Figure 29.1 Parts of the stomach

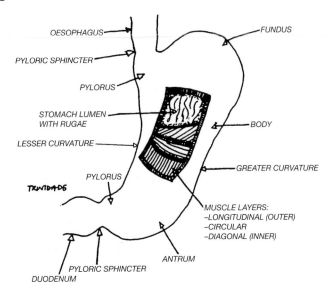

OESOPHAGUS

PYLORIC SPHINCTER

PYLORUS

STOMACH LUMEN
WITH RUGAE

LESSER CURVATURE

PYLORUS

TRINIDADS

DUODENUM

PYLORIC SPHINCTER

ANTRUM

MUSCLE LAYERS:
–LONGITUDINAL (OUTER)
–CIRCULAR
–DIAGONAL (INNER)

GREATER CURVATURE

BODY

FUNDUS

Transverse mesocolon
Splenic artery
Abdominal aorta
Coeliac trunk and branches
Coeliac ganglion
Coeliac lymph nodes
Diaphragm (left crus and dome).
These structures are covered by the
lesser sac which lies between them
and the posterior wall of the stomach.

**What is the entry point to
the lesser sac called?**

The **epiploic foramen** (syn.
foramen of Winslow). Its boundaries
are:
Floor: 1st part of duodenum (D1)
Roof: caudate lobe of the liver
Posterior wall: IVC.
Anterior wall: right free margin of
lesser omentum, which contains:
• Portal vein
• Hepatic artery
• Common bile duct.

What is a hiatus hernia?	A herniation of part of the stomach through the oesophageal hiatus of the diaphragm.
Who does it affect?	M=F; more common in Western societies.
What types do you know of?	**Sliding** and **rolling**.
What is the difference?	**Sliding:** the gastro-oesophageal junction 'slides' upwards into the thorax. Thought to be one of the contributing factors to GORD (see above). **Rolling:** the gastro-oesophageal junction remains in the intra-abdominal cavity, but the stomach **fundus** herniates through the hiatus alongside the distal oesophagus. There is a risk of fundal strangulation. (Syn. **para-oesophageal hernia**). See Figure 29.2.

Figure 29.2 Hiatus hernia

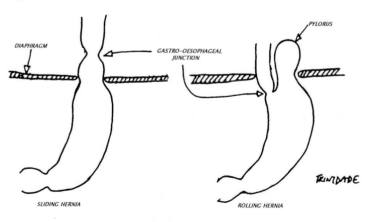

How does it present?	Usually asymptomatic. Pt. may present with symptoms of GORD (*not* necessarily present). Rarely, pts. with large herniae may c/o dysphagia. Equally as rare are pts. with a rolling hernia who present with epigastric pain and signs of strangulation.
What is found on examination?	Often nothing.
What are the investigations?	**Barium meal** is usually diagnostic. Herniation is visualised. If GORD is also present, an OGD is indicated.
What is the treatment?	Sliding hernia may be treated **conservatively** in a similar way to GORD (see above). **Surgical:** especially if GORD is present. Involves oesophageal lengthening (where gastro-oesophageal junction is mobilised and returned to intra-abdominal compartment) and a Nissen's fundoplication (can all be done laparoscopically).
What is Saint's triad?	A triad of three pathologies that have been observed to occur together: 1. Gallstones 2. Hiatus hernia 3. Diverticular disease.

GASTRITIS

What is gastritis?	Inflammation of the stomach mucosal lining resulting in mucosal erosions and ulceration without permanent damage.
What types of gastritis do you know of?	Acute and chronic.

What are the causes of acute gastritis?	Two main causes: 1. Stress, caused in turn, by the following: • Severe burns (Curling's ulcers) • Brain damage (Cushing's ulcers) • Sepsis • Prolonged intubation • Trauma • Shock. 2. Direct insults: alcohol, NSAIDs.
How does acute gastritis present?	As epigastric pain +/− haematemesis (frank or coffee ground).
What is the main differential?	Peptic ulcer disease (PUD).
How do the ulcers in gastritis differ from those in PUD?	They are **multiple, reversible** and do not extend to the **muscularis propria**.
What types of chronic gastritis do you know of?	Type A and Type B.
What is Type A gastritis?	Gastritis associated with **parietal cell antibodies** and **reduced acid production**. There is a genetic predisposition.
What autoimmune disease is Type A gastritis associated with?	Pernicious anaemia (vitamin B_{12} deficiency). (***Mnemonic:*** Type **A** gastritis is **A**utoimmune causing **A**naemia and ↓**A**cid.)
Why?	Parietal cells produce **intrinsic factor** (IF) which is responsible for vitamin B_{12} absorption in the terminal ileum.
What is Type B gastritis?	Chronic gastritis of the **pylorus**, associated with: • Duodenogastric reflux • Chronic alcohol ingestion • Smoking • Gastric surgery.

233

What is the surgical importance of chronic gastritis?	Progression to gastric carcinoma.
How is gastritis diagnosed?	Oesophagogastroduodenoscopy (OGD) with biopsy.
How is it managed?	Antacids and avoidance of precipitating factors.

PEPTIC ULCER DISEASE (PUD)

| **What types of peptic ulcers do you know of?** | Duodenal and gastric ulcers. |
| **Can you compare the two?** | See Table 29.2. |

Table 29.2

	Duodenal ulcer	**Gastric ulcer**
Incidence	0.8% population	0.2% population
Age	40–65 (younger than gastric ulcers)	40–70
Sex	M > F	M > F
Aetiology	• ***Helicobacter pylori* (90–100%)** • Male gender • Smoking • NSAIDs • Zollinger–Ellison syndrome • Hypercalcaemic states: alcoholic cirrhosis, CRF, COPD, hyper-parathyroidism • Familial	• ***Helicobacter pylori* (70–75%)** • Male gender • Alcohol • Smoking • NSAIDs • **Steroids** • Advanced age • Severe illness
Presentation	**Symptoms:** Epigastric pain (pt. points to epigastrium: **pointing sign**), nausea, vomiting. May present with bleeding symptoms: haematemesis (frank or coffee-ground) or melaena stool	

Table 29.2 (continued)

	Duodenal ulcer	**Gastric ulcer**
	Pain relieved by eating and occurs mostly at night (classically biscuits and milk at bedside)	Pain aggravated by eating, and more associated with weight loss and iron deficiency anaemia
	Signs: not many elicited on examination **Abdomen:** epigastric tenderness **DRE:** melaena stool	
Underlying pathology	↑ gastric acid production (esp. in hypercalcaemia states as Ca stimulates gastrin production)	↓ cytoprotection of stomach lining from acid (2ry to ↓bicarbonate and/or mucous production)
Location	Majority are within 2 cm of pylorus in the duodenal bulb	Majority (70%) on lesser curvature of stomach; 5% on greater curvature
Investigation	1. Oesophagogastroduodenoscopy (gold standard): perform **biopsy of ulcer edge** in **gastric** ulcers as these are at ↑ risk of **stomach cancer**. 2. Tests for *H. pylori*: • Blood for antibodies • Urea breath test (*H. pylori* produces **urease** which splits urea, releasing ammonia; test shows ↓urea levels) • Clo test on mucosal biopsy • Microscopy of mucosal biopsy for organisms	
Treatment	**Medical:** symptomatic and antibacterial (against *H. pylori*): Use **CMO regime** (**C**larithromycin, **M**etronidazole, **O**meprazole), 2 antibiotics and a PPI for 1 week. After, continue to use PPIs or H_2-blockers (eg ranitidine)	

Table 29.2 (continued)

	Duodenal ulcer	Gastric ulcer
	Surgical: in the following situations: **mnemonic: I CHOP** **I**ntractability (medical Mx has failed) **C**ancer (gastric ulcers only) **H**aemorrhage (see Chapter 13) **O**bstruction (gastric outlet obstruction 2ry to scarring/stricture formation) **P**erforation (see Chapter 15) The available procedures are listed here, and illustrated below	
	Principle: to reduce acid secretion by dividing the vagus nerve • Truncal vagotomy and pyloroplasty • Selective vagotomy and pyloroplasty • Highly selective vagotomy	**Principle:** to remove the ulcer with the gastrin secreting zone of the antrum • Billroth I partial gastrectomy • Billroth II polya gastrectomy • Vagotomy, pyloroplasty and excision of ulcer • Vagotomy, antrectomy and Roux-en-Y reconstruction

What is _H. pylori_?	A microaerophilic, Gram –ve, urease-forming spiral bacterium which is found normally in the gastric mucosa. It forms an alkaline environment by splitting urea into ammonia.
What type of ulcer is it responsible for?	Duodenal ulcers.
What about gastric ulcers?	Probably (postulated).
What types of ulcer surgery do you know of?	See Figures 29.3 and 29.4.

Figure 29.3 Duodenal ulcer surgery

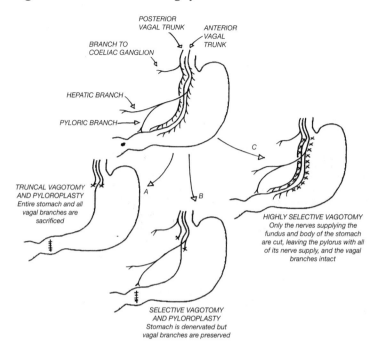

What is a pyloroplasty?	Widening of the diameter of the pyloric inlet. A horizontal incision is made down to, *but not breaching*, the mucosa, and then sutured close in a vertical fashion (see Figure 29.5 below).
Why is a pyloroplasty needed if a vagotomy is done?	The vagus nerve supplies the pylorus which drains the stomach; denervating it causes gastric stasis. Pyloroplasty serves to widen the diameter of the pyloric inlet and hence facilitate drainage.
Why is one *not* done in highly selective vagotomy?	All of the trunks of the vagus nerve are divided *except* the trunk supplying the pylorus (**nerve of Latarjet**).

Figure 29.4 Gastric ulcer surgery

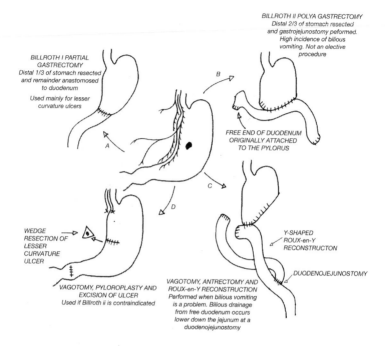

BILLROTH II POLYA GASTRECTOMY
Distal 2/3 of stomach resected and gastrojejunostomy peformed. High incidence of bilious vomiting. Not an elective procedure

BILLROTH I PARTIAL GASTRECTOMY
Distal 1/3 of stomach resected and remainder anastomosed to duodenum
Used mainly for lesser curvature ulcers

B

FREE END OF DUODENUM ORIGINALLY ATTACHED TO THE PYLORUS

A

C

D

WEDGE RESECTION OF LESSER CURVATURE ULCER

Y-SHAPED ROUX-en-Y RECONSTRUCTON

DUODENOJEJUNOSTOMY

VAGOTOMY, PYLOROPLASTY AND EXCISION OF ULCER
Used if Billroth ii is contraindicated

VAGOTOMY, ANTRECTOMY AND ROUX-en-Y RECONSTRUCTION
Performed when bilious vomiting is a problem. Bilious drainage from free duodenum occurs lower down the jejunum at a duodenojejunostomy

What is gastric outlet obstruction?

A chronic complication of long-standing PUD. It involves **cicatrisation** (scarring) of the stomach with resultant severe narrowing of part of the stomach lumen. The following patterns are recognised:

Pyloric stenosis: cicatrisation at the pylorus

Hourglass stomach: cicatrisation around a saddle-shaped lesser curvature ulcer (occurs almost exclusively in women; think hourglass figure!)

Teapot stomach: cicatrisation around a lesser curvature ulcer

Figure 29.5 Pyloroplasty

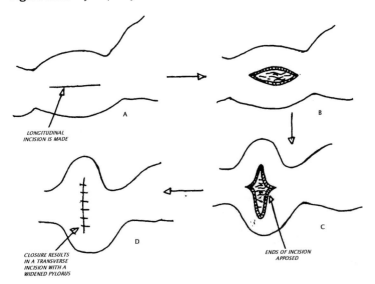

A
LONGITUDINAL
INCISION IS MADE

B

C
ENDS OF INCISION
APPOSED

D
CLOSURE RESULTS
IN A TRANSVERSE
INCISION WITH A
WIDENED PYLORUS

Pyloric stenosis: cicatrisation at the pylorus

Hourglass stomach: cicatrisation around a saddle-shaped lesser curvature ulcer (occurs almost exclusively in women; think hourglass figure!)

Teapot stomach: cicatrisation around a lesser curvature ulcer causing shortening of that stomach border.

ZOLLINGER–ELLISON SYNDROME (ZES)

What is ZES?	A syndrome of gastrin-induced gastric acid overproduction leading to PUD, caused by a **gastrinoma** of the pancreas.
How common is it?	*Rare!*

Does it occur as a single tumour?	No, there tends to be multiple metastases to the surrounding tissue, including the duodenum.
How does it present?	Exactly like PUD, but with a higher incidence of **multiple ulceration** and **intractability**. It may also present as any of the complications of PUD.
What tends to suggest ZES?	Multiple ulcers and ulcers occurring outside the stomach or duodenal bulb.
What percentage of the gastrinomas are malignant?	60% at time of presentation.
How do you investigate for it?	**Blood investigations:** fasting serum gastrin levels **Special investigations:** pentagastrin secretion study **Imaging:** USS or CT scan.
What is the treatment?	**Medical:** as for PUD with PPI (anti-*H. pylori* not necessary) **Surgical:** resection of gastrinoma if localised; if diffuse, metastatic or poorly defined, then surgery as per PUD (vagotomy and pyloroplasty or total gastrectomy).
What other syndrome is ZES associated with?	MEN Type I syndrome.

c. SMALL BOWEL

APPLIED ANATOMY

What are the parts of the small bowel?	Duodenum, jejunum and ileum.
How do you distinguish between jejunum and ileum at laparotomy?	See Table 29.3.

Table 29.3

	Jejunum	Ileum
Length (approx. 20 ft. [610 cm] in total)	Approx. 8 ft.	Approx. 12 ft.
Wall	Thick and double-walled (mucosa can be felt as a separate layer: 'shirt sleeve through a coat sleeve')	Thin and single walled
Colour	Paler	Darker (as richer blood supply)
Vascular arcades (mesenteric arterial loops)	1–2 arcades seen	3–5 arcades seen
Peyer's patches (lymphoid follicles on antimesenteric border)	Sparse	Numerous

What special functions does the ileum have?
1. Absorption of Vitamin B_{12} (intrinsic **terminal** factor dependent)
2. Absorption of bile salts (forms part of the enterohepatic circulation).

What benign tumours occur in the small bowel?
1. Leiomyoma (most common)
2. Lipoma
3. Lymphangioma
4. Haemangioma
5. Fibroma
6. Adenoma.

For conditions of the small bowel (SBO, IBD, herniae), and for carcinoma, see relevant chapters.

d. LIVER

What are the lobes of the liver?

It has four lobes: right, left, quadrate and caudate. The large right lobe is separated from the smaller left lobe by a deep fissure. The quadrate and caudate lobes are seen posteriorly.

What attaches the liver to the diaphragm and anterior abdominal wall?

The falciform ligament.

What is unique about the liver?

It has 2 afferent blood supplies: hepatic artery and portal vein, both of which enter the liver via the porta hepatis.

What is the porta hepatis?

Central region of liver (posterior surface) which contains the hepatic artery, portal vein, lymphatic vessels, and extrahepatic bile ducts.

What structures does the portal vein drain?

Small and large intestines, stomach, spleen, pancreas, and gallbladder.

What is a porto-systemic shunt?

An anatomical area where the portal system (portal vein and tributaries) and the systemic system (IVC and tributaries) anastomose.

Where do you know these to occur?

6 sites in all:
1. Umbilical vein (normally obliterated in the adult where it is known as the **ligamentum teres** or **round ligament** which runs in the free edge of the falciform ligament; anastomoses with epigastric v. [systemic])
2. Gastro-oesophageal junction
3. Retroperitoneal vv.
4. Diaphragmatic vv.

5. Rectal plexus (superior [portal] vv. to middle and inferior [systemic] vv.)
6. Splenic vv. (portal to the short gastric vv. [systemic]).

What are the liver's functions?

They are as follows:
1. Formation of proteins such as albumin prothrombin and fibrinogen
2. Formation of bile, and bilirubin metabolism
3. Metabolism and storage of carbohydrates
4. Metabolism of fats and phospholipids
5. Metabolism of amino acids with the formation of urea
6. Storage of Vitamins B_{12} & A, iron and copper
7. Detoxification and drugs and hormones.

(By knowing the function of the liver well, you can predict the signs/symptoms and blood test changes that may occur in liver damage or failure!)

What are the causes of hepatomegaly?

mnemonic: **CHARM TIPS**
Cirrhosis:
• Alcoholic
• Hepatitis B & C
• Haemochromatosis
• Wilson's disease
• α-1 antitrypsin disease
• Primary biliary cirrhosis.
Congestive cardiac failure
Haematological:
• Thalassaemia
• Sickle cell disease
• Leukaemia
• Lymphoma
• Polycythaemia.

243

Amyloidosis
Reye's syndrome/**R**iedel's lobe
(anatomical variant extending to RIF)
Metabolic:
- Gaucher's disease
- Glycogen storage disease
- Galactosaemia.

Tumour:
- Benign liver tumours
- Hepatocellular carcinoma
- Liver metastases.

Infection:
- Viral: hepatitis (all strains), infectious mononucleosis (EBV), CMV
- Bacterial: hepatic abscess
- Protozoal: malaria, schistosomiasis (kala-azar), leptospirosis (Weil's disease), hydatid cyst.

Portal hypertension/**P**olycystic disease
Sarcoidosis.

PORTAL HYPERTENSION

What is portal hypertension?	Defined as a portal pressure gradient of 12 mmHg or greater and is often associated with varices and ascites. (Normal portal pressure 6–10 mmHg).
What are the two main factors in the development of portal HTN?	1. ↑ vascular resistance (2ry to liver disease) 2. ↑ portal blood flow (2ry to release of endogenous vasodilators).
What are the causes?	Causes divided into **prehepatic, hepatic** and **post-hepatic.** *All* cause ↑ vascular resistance. (The causes are many; say the ones in bold print if nothing else!)

- **Prehepatic: portal vein involvement**
  - **Portal vein thrombosis**
  - **Splenic vein thrombosis**
    - Congenital atresia or stenosis of portal vein
  - Extrinsic compression (tumours)
  - Splanchnic arteriovenous fistula
- **Intrahepatic: liver parenchyma involvement**
  - **Hepatic cirrhosis**
  - **Schistosomiasis**
  - Primary biliary cirrhosis
  - Myeloproliferative diseases (direct infiltration by malignant cells)
  - Polycystic disease
  - Hepatic metastasis
  - Granulomatous diseases (sarcoidosis, tuberculosis
  - Acute and fulminant hepatitis
  - Congenital hepatic fibrosis
  - Vitamin A toxicity (causes non-cirrhotic portal fibrosis)
  - Veno-occlusive disease
- **Posthepatic: IVC involved**
  - **Budd–Chiari syndrome**
  - **Inferior vena cava (IVC) obstruction**
  - **Right heart failure**
  - Constrictive pericarditis
  - Tricuspid regurgitation
  - Arterial-portal venous fistula.

Which liver disease is the most common cause of portal HTN in the UK?	Cirrhosis from any cause.
And worldwide?	Schistosomiasis.
What is Budd–Chiari syndrome?	Thrombosis of the hepatic veins, usually caused by a clotting abnormality.

What are the important points in the history?	1. To determine the **cause**: risk factors for cirrhosis of the liver are the most pertinent.
	2. To determine **complications** of portal HTN:
	   a. Haematemesis or PR bleed (**variceal bleeding**)
	   b. Mental status changes (**portosystemic encephalopathy** due to toxins by-passing failing liver unmetabolised via shunts [see below])
	   c. Abdominal distension (**ascites**)
	   d. Abdominal pain and fever (**spontaneous bacterial peritonitis**).

Where do varices occur?	At portosystemic shunt sites (see anatomy section above). ↑ portal vascular resistance causes backflow of portal blood into systemic system via these shunts. Dilation at these shunt sites are termed varices (sing. **varix**).
How do they present clinically?	In the following ways: **Oesophageal varices:** haematemesis and/or melaena (see Chapter 29a). **Rectal plexus varices:** may cause PR bleed but *not* haemorrhoids (see Chapter 30b). **Umbilical vein:** caput medusa.
What are the clinical findings in portal HTN?	They consist of those of portal HTN itself, and of liver disease: **Portal HTN:** varices (see above) and **splenomegaly** (2ry to splenic congestion; this leads to **hypersplenism** [hyperfunctioning spleen]). **Liver disease:**

General: cachexia, jaundice
Hands: clubbing, palmar erythema, spider naevi, Dupuytren's contracture, liver flap
Face: bilateral parotid enlargement
Chest: gynaecomastia (males), abnormal hair distribution, spider naevi
Abdomen: distension, ascites, hepato-splenomegaly, caput medusa
Genitalia: testicular atrophy.

What do testicular atrophy, gynaecomastia and spider naevi have in common?

All caused by ↑ oestrogen 2ry to ↓ breakdown by failing liver.

What are the investigations?

These are geared mainly towards finding the primary insult (usually cirrhosis).

Blood investigations:
1. FBC: anaemia of chronic disorder and thrombocytopaenia (2ry to hypersplenism)
2. LFTs: ↑AST, ALT, ALP, ↓albumin
3. Clotting screen: ↓ due to ↓clotting factor synthesis (Factors II, VII, IX, X)
4. Viral serology for hepatitis B & C
5. Fe indices (haemochromatosis)
6. Caeruloplasmin level (Wilson's disease)
7. Antinuclear, anti-smooth muscle and anti-mitochondrial antibodies (1ry biliary cirrhosis).

Imaging:
1. **USS:** portal blood flow, splenomegaly, collateral circulation (2ry to portal outflow obstruction).
2. **CT/MRI:** only when USS is inconclusive
3. **Endoscopy:** screening for oesophageal varices.

What is treatment aimed towards in portal HTN?	Bleeding varices. Portal HTN itself is not primarily treated.

BENIGN LIVER TUMOURS

What benign liver tumours do you know of?	1. **Haemangioma**: affects the blood vessels 2. **Hepatocellular adenoma**: arises from hepatocytes 3. **Focal nodular hyperplasia.**
Which is the most common?	Haemangioma (7% of healthy population).
What is it?	A benign vascular tumour of the liver.
Who gets them?	Mainly women (F:M = 6:1); female hormones promote growth.
How do they present?	Mostly asymptomatic and picked up **incidentally** on imaging for other purposes, but if large, may cause RUQ pain.
What is the big risk?	Haemorrhage.
What cardiac complication is it sometimes associated with?	Congestive cardiac failure 2ry to large arteriovenous shunting.
What syndrome is it associated with?	Osler–Weber–Rendu syndrome (amongst other rarer ones!): characterised by numerous small hemangiomas of the face, nares, lips, tongue, oral mucosa, gastrointestinal tract, and liver.
How is it diagnosed?	USS or CT scan with IV contrast. Tagged RBC scan can also be used.
What should *never* be done?	Biopsy! Risk of haemorrhage.
What is the treatment?	Observation. Resect only if symptomatic.

What are the risk factors for hepatocellular adenoma?	1. Female sex (F:M = 9:1, age 15–45) 2. Drugs: OCP and anabolic steroids 3. Glycogen storage disease type 1.
How does it present?	RUQ fullness/tenderness or, rarely, bleeding (7%).
Is there a risk of cancer?	**Yes.** Hepatocellular carcinoma (1%).
How is it diagnosed?	CT/USS +/– biopsy.
What is the treatment?	Stop above drugs; resection.
What is the main differential?	Focal nodular hyperplasia.
How does focal nodular hyperplasia differ from hepatocellular adenoma?	1. The only risk factor is being female 2. No cancer risk 3. CT shows mass with **central scar** 4. Technetium-99 shows it up (but not adenoma) 5. **Histology shows *no* bile ducts whereas adenoma *does*.**
What is the treatment?	Resection if symptomatic (usually pain).

e. BILIARY TREE

APPLIED ANATOMY

What are the parts of the biliary tree?	See Figure 29.6.
What does the common bile duct (CBD) drain into?	2nd part of the duodenum (D2) via the ampulla of Vater (a raised mound on the inner surface of the mid-portion of D2).
What controls bile release into the duodenum at the ampulla?	The sphincter of Oddi.
What is the blood supply of the gallbladder?	The cystic artery, a branch of the right hepatic artery.

Figure 29.6 Biliary tree

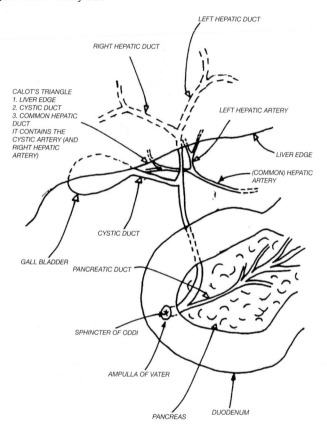

LEFT HEPATIC DUCT

RIGHT HEPATIC DUCT

CALOT'S TRIANGLE
1. LIVER EDGE
2. CYSTIC DUCT
3. COMMON HEPATIC DUCT
IT CONTAINS THE CYSTIC ARTERY (AND RIGHT HEPATIC ARTERY)

LEFT HEPATIC ARTERY

LIVER EDGE

(COMMON) HEPATIC ARTERY

CYSTIC DUCT

GALL BLADDER

PANCREATIC DUCT

SPHINCTER OF ODDI

AMPULLA OF VATER

PANCREAS

DUODENUM

What is Calot's triangle?

An anatomical landmark for the cystic artery, and possibly the right hepatic artery on its way to the liver. Its boundaries are:
1. The common hepatic duct
2. The cystic duct
3. The inferior edge of the liver.

What else is in Calot's triangle?

A lymph node (Calot's node).

What is Hartmann's pouch?	The infundibulum of the gallbladder (ie the portion of the gallbladder that meets the cystic duct).
What is its significance?	It is the most common site of gallstone impaction.
Which liver enzyme is released by the biliary tree?	Alkaline phosphatase (ALP); hence it is raised in biliary tree disease.
What does the gallbladder produce?	Mucus (*not bile!*).

GALLSTONES

What is the function of the gallbladder?	To store and concentrate bile produced by the liver.
What is bile?	A mixture of cholesterol, bile acids, bilirubin and lecithin (a phospholipid).
What is its function?	1. The emulsification of fats. This aids their digestion. 2. The excretion of bile pigments 3. Neutralisation of stomach contents reaching the small bowel.
What causes its release?	Cholecystokinin (CCK), released by the pancreas. Also vagal input.
What stimulates CCK release?	Fats, protein, amino acids and gastric acid in the gut.
How is bile recycled?	Via the enterohepatic circulation. Secreted bile acids are reabsorbed at the terminal ileum and returned to the liver.
What is the formation of gallstones called?	Cholelithiasis.
What type of gallstones do you know of?	Three main types: 1. **Cholesterol stones (20%):** formed by cholesterol supersaturation in bile; risk

factors are hypercholesterolemic states (pregnancy, high cholesterol, diabetes and OCP use).

2. **Pigment stones (5%):** formed in the presence of excess bile pigments; risk factors include haemolytic anaemias (esp. sickle cell disease).

3. **Mixed stones (75%):** mixture of cholesterol and bile.

Who classically get gallstones?

The patient with the **6 Fs**:
Fat
Female
Fair
Fertile
Flatulent
Forty-plus.
(However, in clinical practice, this will hardly be the case!)

How can the potential risks of gallstones be remembered?

Simply by tracing the gallstone's course down the biliary tree:
Gallbladder → Hartmann's pouch/cystic duct → CBD → ampulla of Vater
It may impact and cause problems at any one of these sites.
Gallbladder: may by asymptomatic or cause biliary colic (see below). Long standing stones may cause **gallbladder carcinoma** (see Chapter 42).
Hartmann's pouch/cystic duct: causes back-up of bile in the gallbladder (bile drainage still possible from the liver via CBD), which irritates its wall, causing first a **chemical cholecystitis**, and later, with superinfection, a **bacterial cholecystitis**.

If gallbladder was empty at time of impaction, mucus continues to be secreted, causing a **mucocele**, which may become infected, forming an **empyema** of the gallbladder (see Chapter 16).

CBD: may be asymptomatic, but may also cause back-up of all formed bile into the blood stream (no drainage possible), resulting in **obstructive jaundice** (see below). Superinfection causes **ascending cholangitis** (see Chapter 16).

Ampulla of Vater: obstructive jaundice may still occur, but pancreatic duct is also blocked, resulting in **gallstone pancreatitis** (see Chapter 17).

Also:

Small bowel: stone enters bowel via an **enterocystic fistula** (*not* through the ampulla of Vater!), and lodges at the ileocaecal junction, causing **gallstone ileus** (see Chapter 16).

What percentage of gallstones are asymptomatic?

80%; usually found incidentally on USS done for other reasons.

What is biliary colic?

Rhythmic pain caused by contraction of the gallbladder against a contained gallstone, or against a stone in the cystic duct.

What aggravates it?

Fatty foods: fats in gut stimulate pancreatic CCK release which causes gallbladder contraction.

How is cholelithiasis diagnosed?

Ultrasound (study of choice).

What is the classic USS sign?

Acoustic shadow caused by the gallstone deflecting sound waves.

What percentage of gallstones are visible on plain film?	Only 10%.
Does the gallbladder become distended if the cystic duct is impacted by a gallstone in cholelithiasis?	*No!*
Why not?	Because cholelithiasis causes scarring of the gallbladder, preventing it from distension.
So what would cause the gallbladder to distend?	Cancer of the head of the pancreas causing bile outflow obstruction (gallbladder is not scarred and hence distendable). This is according to **Courvoisier's Law**.
What is Courvoisier's Law?	*If, in the presence of jaundice, the gallbladder is distended, it is unlikely to be due to stones.* (In other words: jaundice + distended gallbladder = cancer of the head of pancreas until proven otherwise. Know this law by heart!)
What is the treatment of a patient with biliary colic?	Cholecystectomy by 1 of 2 methods: **Laparoscopic cholecystectomy:** standard treatment (syn. **lap chole**). **Open cholecystectomy:** via Kocher's incision (see p. 27). Most open choles these days are conversions of failed lap choles.
When would a lap chole be done in an asymptomatic patient?	In the following situations: 1. Sickle cell disease 2. Child with gallstones 3. Porcelain gallbladder (pre-malignant condition; see Chapter 42) 4. Large gallstones > 2–3 cm (risk of gallstone ileus).
What is jaundice?	A serum bilirubin level of >2.5 mg/dl.

How do gallstones cause jaundice?

By obstructing bile outflow due to obstruction of the biliary tree: **obstructive jaundice**.

What is the presence of gallstones in the biliary tree called?

Chole**docho**lithiasis.

How does obstructive jaundice present?

With the following classic symptoms:
1. Jaundice (look at sclerae and under tongue)
2. Pruritis (itching; 2ry to bile salts in skin)
3. Dark urine (2ry to urobilinogen)
4. Clay-coloured (acholic) stools (2ry to absence of stercobilinogen in gut)
5. Nausea
6. Loss of appetite.

Is USS good in diagnosing this?

Not as good as diagnosing cholelithiasis.

Besides USS, what other tests would you do?

The following:
1. **Endoscopic Retrograde Cholangiopancreatography (ERCP):** endoscope is passed down to D2 and sphincter of Oddi is cannulated; dye is injected up biliary tree in a retrograde (backward) fashion, visualising it. Test of choice. May cause pancreatitis.
2. **Percutaneous Transhepatic Cholangiogram (PTC):** hepatic bile ducts are cannulated percutaneously under radiological guidance and dye is injected in an anterograde (forward) fashion. Hepatic vasculature are at risk.
3. **Intraoperative Cholangiogram (IOC):** biliary tree cannulated at operation (lap or open) and dye injected.

What blood investigation *must* be done in a patient with obstructive jaundice pre-op?

Clotting screen: hepatic function may be altered if jaundice is long-standing, causing ↓ production of clotting factors II, VII, IX and X and hence bleeding tendency.

What is the management?

2 modalities:

Minimally invasive: via ERCP; a **sphincterotomy** (division of sphincter of Oddi) is performed to allow passage of stone, or stone retrieval is attempted with a Dormia basket.

Operative: exploration of the CBD with direct stone removal either via lap chole or open. If open, a T-tube is left in situ to allow bile drainage while bile duct heals, thus preventing bile leakage and chemical peritonitis (see Chapter 3 for details on T-tubes).

Is choledocholithiasis the only cause of obstructive jaundice?

No.

What else causes it?

As with any tubular structure, group causes into extraluminal, mural and intraluminal:

Extraluminal:
• Pancreatitis (see Chapter 17)
• Carcinoma head of pancreas (see Chapter 40)
• Pancreatic pseudocyst (see Chapter 17)
• Hepatocellular carcinoma (see Chapter 41)
• Mirizzi syndrome (see below)
• Klatskin tumour (see below).

Mural:
• Cholangiocarcinoma (see Chapter 42)
• Sclerosing cholangitis (see Chapter 16)

- Post-inflammatory stricture
- Post-surgical stricture
- Benign bile duct tumour
- Ampulla of Vater dysfunction.

Intraluminal:
- Choledocholithiasis
- Parasites.

What is Mirizzi's syndrome?	Large gallstone in the cystic duct causing external compression of the common hepatic duct.
What is a Klatskin tumour?	A tumour occurring at the junction of the right and left hepatic ducts causing obstruction and resultant jaundice.
What is a strawberry gallbladder?	A gallbladder whose mucosa is studded with cholesterol deposits in hypercholesterolemia. The inside resembles a strawberry.
What is a porcelain gallbladder?	A gallbladder which has become calcified 2ry to chronic cholelithiasis or cholecystitis. There is a strong cancer risk (see Chapter 42).

f. PANCREAS

APPLIED ANATOMY

Where is the pancreas located?	In the retroperitoneum, forming part of the stomach bed.
What are the parts?	Head, uncinate process, neck, body, tail.
What is the blood supply?	Mainly from the splenic a., but also contributions from the sup. and inf. pancreaticoduodenal aa. (head); venous drainage via splenic v. (drains into portal v.)
What are its functions?	It is both an exocrine and endocrine gland.

Exocrine: produces pancreatic juice containing **trypsin**, **lipase**, and **amylase** (acinar glands) which aids in digestion.
Endocrine: produces glucagon (α-cells) and insulin (β-cells) from the islets of Langerhans located in the tail.

INSULINOMA

What is an insulinoma?

Solitary tumour of the insulin-producing β-cells of the islets of Langerhans. It is the most common islet cell tumour.

How does it present?

Classically with **Whipple's triad:**
1. Low blood sugar level
2. Clinical hypoglycaemia: altered sensorium, vasomotor instability
3. Resolution of symptoms on administration of glucose.

What are the investigations?

Blood investigations:
1. Blood glucose: hypoglycaemia
2. Plasma insulin levels: raised.
Special tests: glucagon test; administered glucagon fails to cause a rise in blood glucose
Imaging: USS, CT scan.

What is the treatment?

Excision, or if tumour cannot be localised, distal pancreatectomy.

Do insulinomas have malignant potential?

Yes.

GLUCAGONOMA

What is a glucagonoma?

Solitary tumour of the Glucagon-producing α-cells of the Islets of Langerhans. Extremely *rare*.

How does it present?	With diabetes and a rash (necrotising migratory erythema).
What is the treatment?	As with insulinomas.

VIPOMA

What is a VIPoma?	A pancreatic tumour which secretes Vasoactive Intestinal Polypeptide, a pancreatic hormone which inhibits gastric acid secretion in normal physiology. It is *rare*. (Syn. **Verner–Morrison syndrome.**)
How does it present?	**W**atery **D**iarrhoea, **H**ypokalaemia, and **A**chlorhydria (hence also known as **WDHA syndrome**).
Why is achlorhydria present?	Due to ↓ gastric acid (HCl) production.
How is it treated?	As with insulinomas.

g. SPLEEN

APPLIED ANATOMY

How can the anatomy of the spleen be remembered?	By the odd numbers 3, 5, 7, 9, 11. Its dimensions are 3 × 5 × 7 inches, and it lies posterior to the 9th to 11th left ribs.
What is its blood supply?	The splenic artery, one of the branches of the coeliac trunk of the abdominal aorta. Venous drainage is to the portal vein via the splenic and left gastroepiploic vv.
What type of organ is it?	A lymphoid organ with the following functions: 1. Filtration of RBCs 2. Platelet storage 3. Opsonin production (important defence against **encapsulated**

organisms, such as *Streptococcus pneumonia*, meningococcus, *Haemophilus influenza* and *Escherichia coli*)
4. Phagocytosis (part of the reticuloendothelial system [RES]).

What are the causes of splenomegaly?

The causes are many:
mnemonic: **CHIASMA**
Congestion:
• Portal hypertension
• Portal/splenic vein thrombosis
• CCF.
Haematological/lymphoreticular:
• Haemolytic anaemia
• Leukaemia
• Myeloproliferative disease (eg multiple myeloma)
• Lymphoma
• Idiopathic thrombocytopenic purpura (ITP)
• Thrombotic thrombocytopenic purpura (TTP).
Infarction (2ry to embolic phenomena):
• Bacterial endocarditis
• Post MI
• Mitral valve stenosis.
Acquired infections:
• Viral: HIV, CMV, infectious mononucleosis (EBV), measles
• Bacterial: TB, typhoid, typhus
• Spirochaetal: syphilis, leptospirosis (Weil's disease)
• Protozoal: malaria, kala-azar.
Storage disease:
• Gaucher's disease.
Masses:
• Cysts: polycystic disease, solitary cysts, hydatid cysts
• Angioma
• Lymphosarcoma.

Autoimmune:

- Rheumatoid arthritis (Felty's syndrome)
- Still's disease
- SLE.

What are the indications for splenectomy?

They include the following:

1. Hypersplenism:
   a. 1ry hypersplenism: abnormal blood elements are removed inappropriately by normal spleen (eg haemolytic anaemia)
   b. 2ry hypersplenism: normal blood elements are removed inappropriately by abnormal spleen (eg portal HTN)
2. Traumatic rupture of the spleen (see Chapter 3)
3. In treatment of splenic abscess or cyst (esp. hydatid)
4. In symptomatic massive splenomegaly (eg myelofibrosis)
5. Incidentally during another surgical procedure (eg radical surgery for gastric cancer)
6. Staging of disease (eg Hodgkin's lymphoma); rarely done now since advent of CT scanning.

What are the complications of splenectomy?

1. Haemorrhage
2. Subphrenic abscess
3. DVT
4. Portal vein thrombosis
5. Overwhelming post-splenectomy sepsis (OPSS)
6. Fistulae (gastric, pancreatic).

What is OPSS?

Sepsis by encapsulated organisms following splenectomy (*S. pneumonia*, meningococcus, *H. influenzae* and *E. coli*).

What should be administered to patients undergoing splenectomy?	**Vaccinations** for *S. pneumonia*, meningococcus and *H. influenzae*. This reduces the risk of OPSS.
What is infectious mononucleosis?	A viral infection caused by EBV. Causes fever, malaise, swollen glands (lymphadenopathy, tonsillitis, splenic enlargement). (Syn. **glandular fever**).
What is the major danger in patients suffering from infectious mononucleosis?	**Traumatic splenic rupture**. Tell patients to avoid contact sports for 2 months.

For the management of splenic rupture, see Chapter 3.

CHAPTER 30: LOWER GASTROINTESTINAL TRACT DISORDERS

a. COLON AND RECTUM

APPLIED ANATOMY

Name the parts of the colon	From proximal to distal: caecum→ascending colon→transverse colon→descending colon→sigmoid colon→rectum.
What are the distinguishing features of the caecum?	The small bowel empties into it via the ileocolic junction (most times guarded by the ileocaecal valve) and it bears the appendix.
How many parts is the rectum divided into?	3, based on their blood supply and venous drainage.
What is the blood supply of the colon?	Mainly branches from the **superior** and **inferior mesenteric arteries** (SMA and IMA respectively): **Caecum:** ileocolic a. [SMA] **Ascending colon:** right colic a. [SMA] **Transverse colon:** middle colic a. [SMA] **Descending colon:** left colic a. [IMA] **Sigmoid colon:** sigmoidal aa. [IMA]
And of the rectum?	**Proximal 1/3:** superior rectal a. (branch of IMA) **Middle 1/3:** middle rectal a. (branch of internal iliac a.) **Distal 1/3:** inferior rectal a. (branch of pudendal a., also a branch of the internal iliac a.).
What is the venous drainage of the colon?	The veins parallel the arteries and have similar names. They all ultimately drain into the **portal vein**.
And of the rectum?	**Proximal 1/3:** inferior mesenteric v.→ splenic v. →portal v. **Middle and distal 1/3:** iliac v. →IVC.

Figure 30.1 Branches of the abdominal aorta

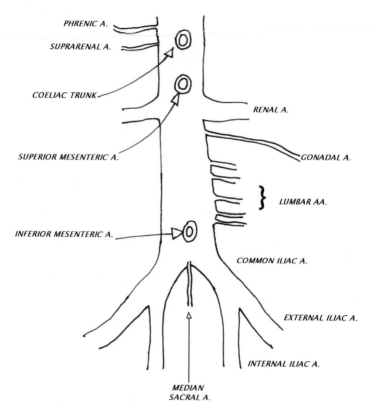

What is the marginal artery of Drummond?	Artery formed by the anastomosis between the ileocolic, middle colic, right and left colic aa., and sigmoidal aa. It is a continuous vessel running along the inner perimeter of the large intestine from the ileocolic junction to the rectum.
What are the features which distinguish the colon from small bowel?	1. Haustrae 2. Taeniae coli 3. Appendices epiploicae (fat appendages)

These are all found on the colon's external surface, whereas the small bowel is smooth and featureless.

COLONIC POLYPS

What is a polyp?

A protuberance of tissue into the lumen of the colon.

Who gets them?

M=F; incidence increases with age.

What are the clinical findings?

Usually nothing, though low polyps may be palpable on rectal exam. Blood may also be present.

How are they usually diagnosed?

On colonoscopy. Biopsy is usually taken at the same time.

What main types of polyps do you know of?

Three main types:
1. Adenomatous
2. Hyperplastic (most common; 90%)
3. Inflammatory.

Of these, which group has malignant potential?

Adenomatous polyps.

Adenomatous polyps

What types of adenomatous polyps do you know of?

Three types:
1. Tubular adenoma (most common; 75%)
2. Villous adenoma
3. Tubulovillous adenoma.

Where in the colon is affected?

Tubular: anywhere
Villous: rectum
Tubulovillous: distal colon and rectum.

Of these, which one has the highest malignant potential?

Villous adenoma: may form **adenocarcinoma.**
mnemonic: think **villainous** adenoma.

How may adenomatous polyps present?

Most are asymptomatic and are found on colonoscopy for other conditions. If symptomatic, they may present as rectal bleeding (with associated anaemia), constipation or diarrhoea.

Which type is famous for diarrhoea?

Villous adenoma, which may cause a hypersecretion syndrome. The diarrhoea is mucoid in nature.

What is usually associated with this diarrhoea?

Hypokalaemia.

What does it look like on colonoscopy?

Classically frond-like projection (like a cauliflower), but can look flat (sessile) with a velvety surface.

How are adenomatous polyps managed?

Solitary may be removed during colonoscopy, potentially curing the patient. In all adenomatous polyps, repeat colonoscopy should be done in 3 years, and then again at 5 years if this is negative.

Hyperplastic and inflammatory polyps

What are hyperplastic polyps?

Totally benign epithelial tumours of the lining of the large bowel with **no malignant potential**.

Where do they mainly occur?

In the rectosigmoid.

What is the treatment?

Resection of solitary ones on colonoscopy is curative. If multiple, biopsy one, and if histology shows hyperplastic polyp, no further management is necessary.

What is an inflammatory polyp?

The type that occurs in ulcerative colitis, more correctly termed a **pseudopolyp**, as it does not have the features of a true polyp.

| **How is it managed?** | It is not managed in isolation, but as part of the treatment of ulcerative colitis (see Chapter 20) which causes resolution. |

POLYPOSIS SYNDROMES

| **What polyposis syndromes do you know of?** | Many! But they can be classified as follows:
 Familial:
 • **Adenomatous familial:**
   1. Familial adenomatous polyposis coli (FAP)
   2. Gardner's syndrome
   3. Turcot's syndrome
 • **Hamartomatous familial:**
   1. Peutz–Jegher's syndrome
   2. Juvenile polyposis syndrome
   3. Cowden syndrome.
 Non-familial: Cronkhite–Canada syndrome |
| **What are their features?** | See Tables 30.1 and 30.2. (If you *must* be selective in which ones you memorise, memorise FAP, Gardner's and Peutz–Jegher's syndromes. The others are asked about less often!) |

Table 30.1

Familial adenomatous polyposis syndromes			
	FAP	**Gardner's syndrome**	**Turcot's syndrome**
Definition	Polyposis of the colon with 100% progression to carcinoma	Polyposis of the colon with 100% progression to carcinoma, with **desmoplastic tendency of fibrous tissue** (variant of FAP)	Polyposis of the colon with almost 100% progression to carcinoma; associated with **brain tumours** (variant of FAP)
Genetics	Autosomal dominant	Autosomal dominant	Autosomal dominant

Table 30.1 (continued)

Demographics	No sex or race difference; polyps by puberty	No sex or race difference; syndrome by age 15–30. Females more prone to developing thyroid cancer	No sex or race difference; symptomatic by 20s
Mortality/ morbidity	Colon cancer develops by age 20–40	Colon cancer develops by age 40	Poor prognosis due to supratentorial brain tumours; death by 20–30
Pathological features	Polyps carpeting the colon, usually starting on the left side. Polyps are 1–2 mm in size	As with FAP, but with the following: Soft tissue tumours GI tumours Bony abnormalities Endocrine tumours Abnormal dentition Medulloblastoma	As with FAP, but with supratentorial gliomas and occasional medullo-blastomas
Clinical features	Vague abdominal pain, PR bleed, diarrhoea	As with FAP but to a lesser extent; obvious path. features (above)	As with FAP but with café-au-lait spots and seizures
Investigations	1. Double contrast barium enema (polyps 1 cm) and colonoscopy (+ve when ⩾ 10 polyps in colon, though close to 100 usually present) 2. Genetic screening for the *APC* gene mutation on chrm 5q (present in 82% of cases) 3. Skin biopsy (Gardner's syndrome)		

Table 30.1 (continued)

Treatment	Subtotal colectomy with ileorectal anastomosis and destruction of any present rectal polyps. *Close follow-up every 6 months for the rest of the patient's life required with subsequent destruction of rectal polyps.* If rectal cancer develops, abdominoperineal resection (removal of rectum and anal canal) with permanent ileostomy is indicated. Alternatively, prophylactic panproctocolectomy can be performed, delaying it until 100 or more polyps occur.
Screening	Annual sigmoidoscopy in 1st degree relatives from puberty (or earlier if symptomatic) until adenomas are found, or they have been proved negative for *APC* gene mutation during genetic screening. If genetic screening not available, annual sigmoidoscopy till age 25, and if no adenomas found, every 2 years till age 35.

Table 30.2

Familial hamartomatous polyposis syndromes			
	Peutz–Jegher's syndrome	**Juvenile polyposis syndrome**	**Cowden syndrome**
Definition	Multiple intestinal hamartomatous polyps associated with mucocutaneous melanotic pigmentation	Familial intestinal hamartomatous polyps (*rare*, but most common polyposis syndrome in kids)	Multiple hamartomatous and neoplastic tumours of ecto-, endo- and mesodermal origin
Genetics	Autosomal dominant	Autosomal dominant	Autosomal dominant
Demographics	No sex or race difference	No race differences; M:F = 3:2	No race difference; mainly affects women
Mortality/ morbidity	40% have non-GI cancers by their 40s. Malignant transformation of polyps is rare.	40% risk of developing colon cancer	50–75% develop breast cancer by their 40s

Table 30.2 (continued)

Pathological features	Multiple hamartomatous GI polyps (not confined to colon; small bowel in 95%) and muco-cutaneous pigmentation, classically of lips, but also occurring on the face and digits. Risk of gonadal tumours	Polyps may occur in colon only, stomach only or entire GIT. Other features include macrocephaly, fibroadenomas and mental retardation	GI polyps together with fibroadenomas and **breast cancer** (often bilateral), bird-like facies, scrotal tongue, skin lesions (papules, keratosis), menstrual irregularities, tremor, seizures
Clinical features	Vague abdominal pain, rectal bleeding and pigmentation; may present with gonadal tumours	Vague abdominal pain, rectal bleeding, rectal prolapse and intussusception together with above features	Variable, and depends on which pathological features are present
Investigations	Double contrast barium enema (polyps >1 cm) and colonoscopy (+ve when ≥ 10 polyps in colon, though close to 100 usually present)		
Treatment	1. See *Treatment* in Table 30.1 2. Prophylactic mastectomy in women with active cystic breast disease in Cowden syndrome		
Screening	**Peutz–Jegher's:** colonoscopy, oesophagogastroduodenoscopy, and small-bowel follow-through studies every 2 years after diagnosis; women should undergo annual mammograms; surveillance of gynaecologic or testicular tumours. **Juvenile polyposis:** colonoscopic examination every 5 years, beginning at age 12 years. For families with familial juvenile polyposis of the stomach, oesophagogastroscopy is substituted for colonoscopy. Patients with polyps should undergo endoscopic surveillance every 1–3 years. **Cowden syndrome:** endoscopic screening *not* necessary; screen for breast disease (mammograms 6–12 monthly) or other affected organs (eg thyroid)		

How can the various features of Gardner's syndrome be remembered?

mnemonic: Think of Gardner walking through the **GARDENS** thinking of his syndrome:

GI tumours:
- Colonic adenomatous polyps
- Duodenal adenomatous polyps (90% chance malignancy)
- Periampullary carcinoma
- Hepatoblastoma
- Pancreatic carcinoma

Abnormal dentition:
- Supernumerary teeth
- Predisposition to caries

Ribs and other bony abnormalities:
- Exostoses (benign, self-limiting bony tumours)

Desmoid tumours

Endocrine tumours:
- Thyroid carcinoma (mainly papillary)
- Carcinoid tumours
- Parathyroid adenomas
- Pituitary adenomas

Nervous system tumours:
- Medulloblastoma

Soft tissue tumours:
- Epidermoid (sebaceous) cysts
- Lipomas
- Fibromas
- Neurofibromas
- Leiomyomas
- (Desmoid tumours are also classified here, but are listed under 'D'!).

Which drug is thought to cause regression of polyps in FAP?

Sulindac (an NSAID).

What is Cronkhite–Canada syndrome?

Generalised GI polyposis with neuroectodermal changes, alopecia, hyperpigmentation and nail atrophy (*extremely rare!*)

What is rectal prolapse?

Emergence of the rectum through the anus. The rectum in effect turns itself inside out.

What types of prolapse do you know of?

1. Complete (full thickness)
2. Incomplete (mucosal)
3. Concealed (internal).

How do they differ?

Complete: involves all the walls of the rectum, and is most common in elderly females. There is usually associated pelvis floor weakness.
Incomplete: only the rectal mucosa prolapses through the anus, and can occur in children and adults. Associated with forcing at stool. Occasionally seen in **cystic fibrosis**.

Concealed: prolapse occurs, but not through the anus. It occurs higher up in the form of an intussusception, usually involving the upper 1/3 of the rectum intussuscepting into the lower 1/3.

Why is complete prolapse more common in females?

Higher incidence of pelvis floor weakness 2ry to trauma at childbirth.

What anatomical defect may predispose to complete prolapse?

Redundant rectosigmoid colon.

How does prolapse present?

The patient complains of a lump at the anus which has occurred spontaneously or after coughing or straining during exertion or at stool. The patient may or may not be able to self-reduce it.
It is often not the first episode. Pruritis ani, bleeding and faecal incontinence are common.

What are the clinical features?	**Complete:** a cylindrical anal mass with a visible lumen, seen as a pit in the centre of concentric circumferential folds of bright red mucosa. It may be reducible (unlikely if oedematous). PR reveals lax anal tone.
	Incomplete: only bright red mucosa seen at anus, resembling prolapsed haemorrhoids (**main differential**).
	Concealed: no obvious anal findings; patient presents with intermittent bouts of crampy lower abdominal pain (in keeping with intussusception) +/– symptoms of obstruction.
What is the management?	**Complete:** patient is usually frail and not a good surgical candidate; self-reduction should be taught in these cases. Otherwise surgery can be performed to correct the prolapse via either a **perineal approach** (eg perineal rectopexy or Delorme's procedure) or an abdominal approach (eg abdominal rectopexy; higher morbidity, less recurrence).
	Incomplete: surgery rarely indicated; dietary advice is important, and intervention is as for haemorrhoids (see later).
	Concealed: Treated as an intussusception with diagnostic/ prophylactic Ba enema to reduce it. If this fails, resection of intussuscepting part is undertaken.

PROCTALGIA FUGAX

What is proctalgia fugax?	Severe, spasmodic rectal pain of unknown aetiology, usually occurring at night.
How long does it last?	Typically a few seconds to several minutes.

What is thought to possibly cause it?	Spasm of the pelvis floor muscles (levator ani). High stress levels are thought to play a role.
Who are more prone to getting it?	Medical students and junior doctors!
What is the history?	Usually of just the pain, but occasionally it is known to follow an episode of forcing stool or ejaculation.
What is the treatment?	None, although inhaled salbutamol has been shown to shorten attacks.

b. ANAL CANAL

APPLIED ANATOMY

How long is the anal canal?	4 cm long.
What is normally palpable on rectal exam?	**Both sexes:** rectal mucosa parasacral lymph nodes (if enlarged) and tip of coccyx **Males:** prostate and seminal vesicles anteriorly **Female:** upper 1/3 of vagina and cervix anteriorly.
What is its blood supply?	**Upper end:** superior rectal a. **Lower end and mucosa:** inferior rectal a. Also receives supply from the middle rectal and median sacral aa.
What is its venous drainage?	**Superior rectal v.**, which drains the upper part and is continuous with the rectal venous plexus, and then on to the inferior mesenteric and portal vv. **Inferior and middle rectal vv.**, which drain the lower part into the internal iliac v. and then on to the IVC. *The anal canal is therefore a site of porto-systemic anastomosis.*

Where does this anastomosis occur?

At the **anal cushions**, spongy mucosal cushions that occur at 3, 7, and 11 o' clock (taken in the lithotomy position).

What else are these anal cushions important for?

They help maintain continence of flatus and keep the anal canal watertight.

What sphincters control the anus?

Internal (under involuntary control) and external (under voluntary control).

What is the nerve supply of

Somatic: inferior rectal branches (S2) of the pudendal n. supply the external sphincter and sensory supply of the lower end of the canal (hence painful conditions of the anus are registered via this nerve, and the external sphincter is under voluntary control).
Autonomic: supply the internal sphincter and upper end.
Sympathetic supply (pelvic plexus) causes contraction and **parasympathetic supply** (pelvis sphlanchnic n.) causes relaxation (hence upper anal canal is **insensate** and under *in*voluntary control).

What anatomical landmark divides the sensory parts of the anal canal?

The **dentate line**: above this line is insensate; below this line is **cutaneous** and registers pain.

What is the dentate line also a landmark for?

The **anal valves**: these contain submucosal glands, some of which penetrate into the internal sphincter. Infection of these glands may result in abscesses (see Chapter 24) +/– fistulae (see later).

What are the ischioanal fossae?

Wedge-shaped, fat-filled spaces on either side of the anal canal (syn. **ischiorectal fossae**, a misnomer).

What are their boundaries?	**Base:** skin over anal region of perineum
	Medial wall: anal canal and levator ani
	Lateral wall: ischial tuberosity below and obturator internus muscle above
	Apex: where the medial and lateral walls meet.
What is their significance?	Site of anorectal abscess formation (see Chapter 24 and fistulae-in-ano later).

HAEMORRHOIDS

What are haemorrhoids?	Enlargement of the anal cushions within the walls of the anus.
What are they also known as?	Internal haemorrhoids or piles.
What causes them?	Straining at stool: the mucosal lining of the anal cushions 'stretch' and become redundant. This redundant mucosa may then prolapse out of the anus, presenting as a lump.
Does portal hypertension cause haemorrhoids?	*No!* There is no evidence that haemorrhoids are caused by portal hypertension.
How do they present?	As a painless (or sometimes painful) bleeding lump from the anus that may or may not spontaneously reduce. There is a history of bright red bleeding per rectum which may be discovered on wiping or covering the stool. There may also be a history of dripping into the bowl. **Faecal soiling** and **pruritis ani** are common.
What is a common point in the history?	Constipation and forcing at stool.

What else predisposes to haemorrhoids?

Pregnancy and straining at labour.

How are haemorrhoids classified?

1ry, 2ry, 3ry, and 4ry:
Primary: bleeding only
Secondary: bleeding and prolapse with spontaneous reduction
Tertiary: bleeding and prolapse that must be manually reduced
Quaternary: bleeding and prolapse that never reduces.

When are haemorrhoids painful?

When anal spasm strangulates a prolapsed pile, causing congestion and oedema. A blood clot may form within the contained venous plexus, resulting in a **thrombosed pile**.

What is the management?

Conservative: analgesia and high residue diet; Sitz baths (sitting in warm salt solution) is thought to give symptomatic relief by reducing oedema by an osmotic effect.
Outpatient: there are two modalities of treatment, usually reserved for 1ry and 2ry haemorrhoids:
1. **Banding:** a rubber band is placed around the haemorrhoid, causing ischaemia and fibrosis (with resultant shrinkage).
2. **Injection sclerotherapy:** 5% phenol in arachis or almond oil is injected into the haemorrhoidal mucosal lining causing sclerosis and shrinkage (beware injecting anterior haemorrhoids in men as inadvertent injection into the prostate gland may cause prostatitis); less effective than banding.

What is important when performing the above outpatient procedures?

Ensuring that you are above the **dentate line** (no pain receptors!).

What are the surgical options?	Reserved for 3ry and 4ry piles: **Haemorrhoidectomy:** small risk of anal stenosis and incontinence; may be done either by an open procedure or via staple technique.
How is the risk of anal stenosis reduced?	By leaving 'bridges' of mucosa between excised piles during haemorrhoidectomy.
What is the most common post-op complication?	**Pain.** Reduced by giving metronidazole (oral or suppository), or Botox injection (intra-op).

FISTULA-IN-ANO

What is a fistula-in-ano?	A hollow tract lined with granulation tissue connecting a primary opening inside the anal canal to a secondary opening in the perianal skin (**external opening**). Secondary tracts may be multiple and from the same primary opening.
What causes it?	Almost always a **previous anorectal abscess** which has tracked down to the perianal skin (see Chapter 24).
What types are there?	Based on the relation of the fistula to the anal sphincters. *mnemonic:* **SITE** (based on the Parks classification system) **S**uprasphincteric (5%) **I**ntersphincteric (70%) **T**rans-sphincteric (25%) **E**xtrasphincteric (<1%) (See Figure 30.2.)

Figure 30.2 Fistula-in-ano

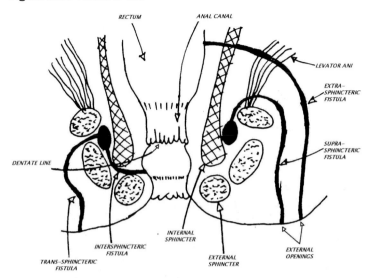

What is Goodsall's rule?	External openings occurring **below** the transverse anal line represent fistulae which track back along a **curved route** to the dentate line in the **midline posteriorly**; those occurring **above** this line track back to the dentate line via a **direct radial route** (see Figure 30.2).
What is the transverse anal line?	An imaginary transverse line drawn through the anus with the patient in the lithotomy position (see Figure 30.3).
How do fistulae-in-ano present?	With one or more of the following: 1. Perianal discharge, usually mucopurulent 2. Perianal lump or (representing an external opening) 3. Itching and soiling 4. Perianal pain 5. Bleeding per rectum.

Figure 30.3 Goodsall's rule

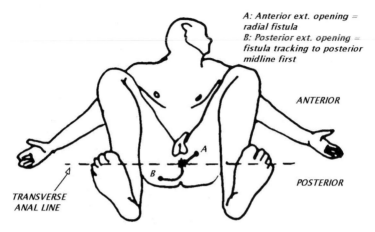

A: Anterior ext. opening = radial fistula
B: Posterior ext. opening = fistula tracking to posterior midline first

ANTERIOR

POSTERIOR

TRANSVERSE ANAL LINE

What are the important points in the history?

1. Previous anorectal abscesses or fistulae
2. Crohn's disease (especially in multiple fistulae or watering can perineum; see Chapter 20)
3. Diverticulitis (see Chapter 19)
4. History of colorectal cancer.

What are the clinical findings?

External openings on inspection (keep Goodsall's rule in mind), and internal openings on rectal examination. There may be visible soiling and discharge from the fistulae, excoriation and scratch marks from pruritis ani. Keep a look out for colorectal cancer on rectal exam.
On general examination, look for evidence of Crohn's disease.

What are the investigations?

Clinical examination is usually enough for first time presentation of a fistula with no other complications. Otherwise:

1. MRI: may be necessary in complex fistulae or fistulae not responding to treatment.
2. Rectal USS: can also be used
3. Examination under anaesthesia (EUA) is sometimes necessary, but is usually done prior to a definitive procedure (see below).

What is the management?

Depends on relation to the sphincter.
Low fistulae: includes submucosal, inter-sphincteric and low trans-sphincteric; fistula is **laid open** by passing a metal probe through the fistula and cutting down onto the probe, and **saucerised** (wide, shallow area is excised, removing all granulation tissue, and allowing healing to occur from the base of the 'saucer' upwards).
High fistulae: includes high trans-sphincteric, suprasphincteric and extrasphincteric; a 2-part procedure is performed:
1. The lower part of the fistula not involving the sphincter is laid open as in low fistulae
2. In the part of the fistula involving the sphincter, a **seton** is applied.

What is a seton?

A suture (usually silk) that is threaded through the remaining part of the fistula. It can be used in 1 of 2 ways:
1. **Cutting through:** the seton is applied **tightly** (and periodically further tightened on visits to the office over 6–8 weeks) in an attempt to gradually cut through the fistula, leaving a path of fibrosis behind it, hence closing off the fistula and leaving the sphincter intact.

2. **Drainage and fibrosis:** the seton is applied **loosely** to promote draining healing of the fistula (2–3 months). During this time, fibrosis occurs in the affected area of the sphincter. This fibrosed area and seton are excised at a later operation leaving the rest of the sphincter intact.

PERIANAL HAEMATOMA

What is a perianal haematoma?	A painful condition caused by rupture of a blood vessel under the skin surrounding the anus.
How does it present?	As a painful anal lump. There may be a history of straining or heavy lifting.
What are the clinical findings?	A tense, tender lump close to, but not usually involving the anus. May be bluish in colour in fair-skinned people due to blood clot.
What is its natural history?	Usually self-resolving with slowly improving symptoms.
What is the treatment?	Usually only symptomatic as they are self-resolving. However, in acutely painful ones, the blood clot can be expressed by incision under local anaesthetic with instant relief. No suturing is required, as they heal well.
What is a perianal haematoma also known as?	An external haemorrhoid (confusing term).

What is a fissure-in-ano?	A tear in the mucosal lining of the anus (syn. **anal fissure**).
What causes it?	Thought to be secondary to anal sphincter spasm which compromises blood supply leading to mucosal ischaemia.
What is its incidence?	M=F.
How does it present?	As severe, spasmodic anal pain, usually aggravated by passage of hard stool. There is a history of bright red blood on wiping after defecation or covering the surface of the stool (as opposed to blood being *mixed in* with the stool as occurs in colorectal cancer). **Pruritis ani** (perianal itching) is also common.
How long is the history?	Usually a chronic history of approximately 6 weeks).
What are the clinical findings?	A tear may be obvious on inspection. Rectal examination is usually **not allowed** due to exquisite tenderness (classic finding!). There may be **skin tags** (known as a **sentinel pile**) due to previously healed fissures.
Which part of the anus is usually affected?	Posterior fissures are by far more common.
Who are more prone to getting anterior fissures?	Women.
Why?	Anterior fissures are more common during labour. (Posterior fissures are *still* more common in women than anterior ones, though.)
What must you suspect in multiple or recurrent fissures?	Crohn's disease and TB.

What is the management?

Conservative: topical anaesthetic agents (eg lignocaine gel) and stool softeners for symptomatic relief and prevention of constipation. **GTN or diltiazem cream** also helps by increasing blood flow to the ischaemic area, hence enhancing healing of the fissure. Treatment course is approximately 6 weeks.

Surgery: reserved for chronic fissures not responding to conservative measures. Options include:

1. **Lateral sphincterotomy:** the **internal** sphincter is divided in an attempt to release spasm and improve blood supply (*not* the external sphincter as incontinence will ensue! Higher risk of incontinence also present if a posterior sphincterotomy is done due to damage to **puborectalis**, the so-called **anal sling**).

2. **Anal dilation (Lord's procedure):** stretching the anus (classically by inserting five fingers into the anus) relieves symptoms. Not commonly done now due to higher risk of incontinence.

Other: botulinum (Botox) injection (chemical sphincterotomy).

CHAPTER 31: VASCULAR DISEASE

a. ARTERIAL DISORDERS

APPLIED ANATOMY

What is the blood supply of the lower limb? See Figure 31.1.

What is the landmark for the (common) femoral artery? Mid-inguinal point (feel here for femoral pulse).

Figure 31.1 Blood supply of the lower limb

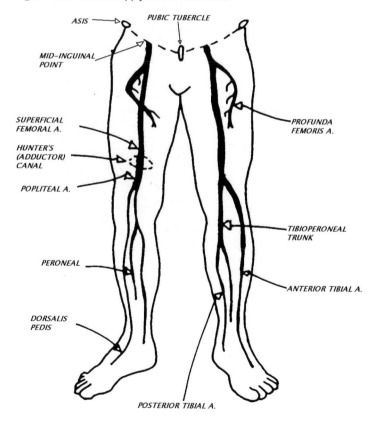

ASIS

PUBIC TUBERCLE

MID–INGUINAL POINT

SUPERFICIAL FEMORAL A.

HUNTER'S (ADDUCTOR) CANAL

POPLITEAL A.

PROFUNDA FEMORIS A.

TIBIOPERONEAL TRUNK

PERONEAL

ANTERIOR TIBIAL A.

DORSALIS PEDIS

POSTERIOR TIBIAL A.

What are the branches of the common femoral artery?

After entering the thigh, it gives off 4 cutaneous aa.:
1. Superficial circumflex iliac a.
2. Superficial epigastric a. (important landmark in the inguinal region!! See p. 285)
3. Superficial external pudendal a.
4. Deep external pudendal a.

It then divides into:
1. **Profunda femoris a.** (supplies the thigh muscles)
2. **Superficial femoral a. (SFA)** which enters the adductor (Hunterian) canal (see below).

What happens to the SFA in the popliteal fossa?

It becomes the **popliteal a.** and then **trifurcates** into:
1. Anterior tibial a.
2. Posterior tibial a.
3. Peroneal a.

What is the popliteal fossa?

A diamond-shaped area behind the knee.

What are its boundaries?

Superio-medially: semi-membranosus and semitendinosus
Superio-laterally: tendon of biceps femoris
Inferio-medially/laterally: medial and lateral heads of gastrocnemius
Roof: fascia lata, pierced by the **saphenous n.**

What pulses are palpable in the foot?

The dorsalis pedis and the posterior tibial.

What are their landmarks?

Dorsalis pedis: at the dorsum of the foot between the extensor hallucis longus and extensor digitorum longus tendons (or the tendons of the big and second toes!)
Posterior tibial: midway along an imaginary line, joining the point of the heel and the medial malleolus.

What is peripheral vascular disease (PVD)?	Chronic ischaemia of lower limb 2ry to atherosclerosis, manifesting clinically along a spectrum of severity: <div align="center">Asymptomatic ↓ Intermittent claudication ↓ Rest pain ↓ Ulceration/gangrene</div>
What is the pathological progression of atherosclerosis?	A **fatty streak** appears in early life in the arterial lumen. This then progresses to a **fibrous plaque,** a cap of smooth muscle cells and connective tissue overlying a core of cholesterol esters. Finally it becomes a **complicated lesion**, where ulceration, haemorrhage, calcification and necrosis occur. This exposes a highly thrombogenic surface leading to platelet activation and formation of a **thrombotic plug**.
What are the risk factors for atherosclerosis?	1. Male sex 2. Smoking 3. Diabetes 4. Hypertension 5. Hyperlipidaemia 6. Family history.
How do you classify chronic limb ischaemia (PVD)?	**The Fontaine Classification**: *Stage I*: asymptomatic *Stage II*: intermittent claudication limiting lifestyle *Stage III*: rest pain *Stage IV*: ulceration/gangrene A patient in stages III & IV is said to have **critical ischaemia**.

What is intermittent claudication?	**Ischaemic muscular pain** brought on by exercise at a reproducible walking distance, and relieved by a period of rest.
	Pain usually in the **calves**, but may also be present in the **buttocks** and **thighs** (**Leriche's syndrome**, caused by **aorto-iliac** disease; also includes **impotence**) depending on the level of occlusion.
	Affects 5% of men over 50 years of age.
What is critical ischaemia?	The presence of **rest pain** (pain in the foot at rest, particularly at night, relieved by hanging foot over edge of bed), **ulceration** or **gangrene** indicates critical limb ischaemia.
	The peak incidence is 70–79 years. 50–100 per 100,000 are affected every year in the UK.
What are the clinical findings in PVD?	**Limbs:** *Inspection:* loss of hair, atrophic nails, dusky peripheries, ulcers in **lateral gaiter region** (lateral aspect of foot). *Palpation:* cool periphery, absent pulses, positive **Buerger's sign** (blanching on limb elevation followed by hyperaemia on hanging over edge of bed), popliteal aneurysms. *Auscultation:* possible bruits, especially over **Hunter's canal** (the site of the **superficial femoral artery [SFA]**, most common site of atherosclerosis)
	General: this *must* be performed. Examine abdomen for AAA, carotids for bruits and perform a full CVS exam. Remember, patients with PVD are usually **atheropaths** (ie they have widespread atherosclerosis).

| **How many patients with a popliteal aneurysm will also have an AAA?** | 50%. |

| **What are the differential diagnoses of claudication?** | 1. Spinal canal stenosis
2. Compartment syndrome
3. Sciatica
4. Venous claudication after extensive iliofemoral DVT. |

How would you investigate symptoms of chronic limb ischaemia?

Blood investigations:
1. FBC: anaemia can mimic/ aggravate
2. RBS: r/o diabetes
3. Lipid profile for hyperlipidaemia.

Non-invasive tests:
1. APBI (see below)
2. Exercise tests to determine exercise tolerance.

Imaging:
1. Duplex ultrasound to determine blood flow
2. Angiography to identify stenotic areas (*only* done in potential surgical candidates due to inherent risks of the procedure)
3. Magnetic resonance angiography (MRA; alternative to angiography).

What is the significance of the Ankle Brachial Pressure Index (ABPI)?

It gives a ratio of the BP distally compared to the systemic BP. Ratios are interpreted as:
Normal = 1, claudication = 0.5, rest pain = 0.3, and impending gangrene ≤ 0.2.

How would you measure it?

Take the ratio of the blood pressure at the dorsalis pedis artery (BP cuff at ankle) and the brachial artery (BP cuff at arm). Use a hand held Doppler probe instead of a stethoscope.

What specific problems do diabetic patients have?

Tendency to have microvascular disease, and more distal atherosclerosis. Vessels are frequently calcified which gives an **artificially high ABPI reading (> 1).**

How would you treat chronic limb ischaemia?

Risk factor modification (includes **cessation of smoking**, drug therapy for diabetic and lipid control), and increasing exercise tolerance.
Surgical intervention only in the following:
1. Rest pain
2. Gangrene
3. Infection
4. Severe claudication refractory to conservative measures.

Interventions include:
1. Angioplasty +/− stenting
2. Bypass surgery, using vein (autologous) or synthetic grafts.

What types of bypasses do you know of?

Anatomical:
Femoro-popliteal (Fem Pop): used to bypass SFA occlusion; graft from femoral a. to popliteal a. (use either autologous or synthetic).
Femoro-distal (Fem Distal): used to bypass more distal occlusions; graft from femoral a. to a distal a., such as peroneal, anterior tibial or posterior tibial aa. (use autologous graft only as high chance of failure with synthetic).
Extra-anatomical:
Axillo-femoral: used if original graft becomes infected; graft goes from axillary a. to the femoral a.
Femoro-femoral (Fem Fem): usually used in conjunction with an axillo-femoral bypass; graft goes from one femoral a. to the other.

What type of grafts do you know of?

Autologous: usually long saphenous vein, which can either be **harvested** and reversed to allow blood flow distally past the valves (**reverse vein graft**), or left *in situ* (***in situ* vein graft**). In the latter, the valves must be destroyed with a valvulotome. **Synthetic:** either Dacron or polytetrafluoro-ethylene (PTFE).

ABDOMINAL AORTIC ANEURYSM

What is an aneurysm?

An abnormal dilation on a blood vessel to more than twice its diameter (if less than twice the diameter, the vessel is said to be ecstatic). An **a**bdominal **a**ortic **a**neurysm (syn. **AAA** or **'triple A'**) is defined as one with a diameter of >3 cm.

What types of AAA do you know of?

Supra-renal (5%) and infra-renal (95%).

What is the incidence?

5% of all patients > 60 years old, and 1 in 5 patients with PVD.

What are the causes of aneurysm formation?

The same for all aneurysms.
mnemonic: **A**neurysms **M**ay **S**ometimes **C**ause **T**errible **B**leeding
Atherosclerosis (most common cause)
Mycotic (2ry to endocarditis [*not* fungal as name suggests!]; occurs at bifurcations)
Syphilitic
Connective tissue disorders (Marfan's syndrome, Ehlers–Danlos syndrome)
Trauma
Berry aneurysm (and other congenital aneurysms).

What types of aneurysms are there?	Can be classified as follows: 1. **True** or **pseudoaneurysm**: true aneurysmal dilation involves all layers of the vessel wall; pseudoaneurysm is caused by trauma with resultant bleed into, and compression by, surrounding tissues (which form the pseudosac). 2. **Fusiform** or **saccular**: fusiform dilation involves entire circumference of the vessel; saccular involves bulging of vessel wall at one point of weakness.
How does an AAA present?	1. Asymptomatic incidental finding on examination or on scanning for other reasons. 2. Pulsatile, expansile mass in the abdomen (commonly the epigastrium) may cause epigastric or back pain (leaking aneurysm) (see Chapter 22). 3. As an emergency ruptured aneurysm (see Chapter 22).
What are the indications for elective surgery?	AAA > 5 cm diameter (as ↑ risk of rupture with ↑ size).
What surgery should be done?	(See Chapter (22).

b. VENOUS DISORDERS

APPLIED ANATOMY

What are the venous tributaries of the lower limb?	See Figure 31.2.

Figure 31.2 Venous tributaries of the lower limb

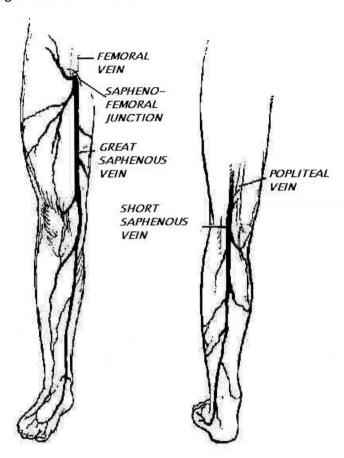

What is the course of the long saphenous vein?

Begins in front of the medial malleolus and travels upwards along medial surface of tibia towards the knee. Passes **1 handsbreadth medial to the patella** and runs up the medial aspect of the thigh. Enters the **cribriform fascia** 3.5 cm below and lateral to the pubic tubercle.

293

What about the short saphenous vein?

Begins behind the lateral malleolus and runs upwards along the surface of the calf to drain into the popliteal v. at the level of the popliteal fossa.

What does the long saphenous vein drain into?

The femoral v. after perforating the cribriform fascia.

At what levels are its perforators?

Long saphenous v.: at 5, 10 and 15 cm above the medial malleolus, at Hunter's canal and at the sapheno-femoral junction (SFJ). **Short saphenous v.:** at the popliteal fossa.

What is the significance of these perforators?

They communicate with the deep venous system via a one-way valve system (blood drains from superficial to deep).

What happens if these valves become incompetent?

There is backflow of blood into the superficial system, ie **varicose veins** (see below).

Where is the sapheno-femoral junction?

Where the saphenous vein dives deep to join the femoral vein, medial to the femoral pulse, or 2 cm below and lateral to the pubic tubercle.

What veins drain at the sapheno-femoral junction (SFJ)?

1. Superficial circumflex iliac v.
2. Superficial epigastric v.
3. Superficial external pudendal v.
4. Deep external pudendal v.

VARICOSE VEINS

What are varicose veins?

Tortuous, distended, thickened veins, usually in the distribution of the long and/or short saphenous veins (the superficial veins of the lower limbs).

What is the prevalence?	Prevalence of **chronic venous insufficiency** in general varies from <1% to 40% in females and from <1% to 17% in males. Prevalence estimates for varicose veins are higher, <1% to 73% in females and 2% to 56% in males.
What causes varicose veins?	Incompetent valves between the deep and superficial systems allow backflow from the higher pressure system to the superficial veins. There is an association with **occlusion of the venous system** by pregnancy, fibroids, pelvic tumour and DVT. Other risk factors are: older age, female gender, family history of venous disease, obesity, and occupations associated with orthostasis (stasis of blood in the lower limbs from standing for long periods).
What is a saphena varix?	A varicosity of the saphenous v. as it joins the femoral v., causing a blue, compressible swelling in the groin, with a cough impulse and a palpable thrill on coughing (the latter is known as **Cruveilhier's sign**) It disappears on lying down. Differential diagnoses include causes of a **groin lump:** femoral hernia, lymph nodes, ectopic testis, psoas abscess and skin lumps.
What are the signs of chronic venous insufficiency?	*mnemonic:* **HEAVE** **H**aemosiderin deposition (2ry to blood stasis) **E**czema (venous) **A**nkle ulcers (over medial gaiter region) **V**aricose veins o**E**dema.

How are varicose veins demonstrated clinically?

Tourniquet test: the limb is elevated and drained of blood. A tourniquet is applied at the level of one of the perforators to occlude it (start with SFJ). The patient is asked to stand up. Repeat test at different perforator levels.
Interpretation: if tourniquet controls refilling of superficial system, then the incompetence is at the level of the occluded perforator. If the tourniquet *doesn't* control refilling, then incompetence is *at least* at the level of the occluded perforator.

What is an alternative to the tourniquet test?

Trendelenburg test: a fingertip is used to occlude perforators at their anatomical landmarks instead of a tourniquet.

What is the investigation of choice for varicose veins?

Duplex ultrasonography: can define direction of blood flow in the vessels, and where the incompetencies lie.

What is the treatment of varicose veins?

Conservative: graded compression stockings.
Minimal intervention: injection with sclerosant; causes endovascular obliteration resulting in venous obstruction by shrinkage of the vein and thrombus formation.
Surgical: high tie of the saphenous v. at the groin (including draining tributaries; see above); stripping of the saphenous to the knee; and stab avulsions over lower varicosities. (Stripping the calf vein risks damage to the saphenous nerve.)

What is the treatment of chronic venous insufficiency?

4 layer compression bandaging, provided that there is no evidence of arterial disease (check ABPI).

What is a DVT?	Deep venous thrombosis, causing a swollen, tense, tender, warm lower limb, with dilated surface veins.
What are the risk factors?	Immobility Hypercoagulable states (protein S or C deficiency) Tumours (esp. pelvic) Smoking ($\uparrow$ risk if on OCP) Previous DVT Surgery in the last 3 months (esp. orthopaedic and gynaecological) Varicose veins Advanced age IV drug use (6.9%).
How does a pulmonary thromboembolism (PE) present?	Sudden collapse (or death) Pleuritic pain Respiratory distress: shortness of breath, cyanosis Shock Haemoptysis. Look for: tachycardia, raised JVP, pleural rub.
Which tests are useful in PE?	ABGs; ECG (tachycardia, right axis deviation, right bundle branch block, $S_1Q_3T_3$ pattern); CXR (pulmonary wedge); spiral chest CT scan; V/Q scan

LEG ULCERS

How do you distinguish different types of leg ulcer?	(See Table 31.1)
What are the other causes of ulceration?	Trauma, malignancy, rheumatoid arthritis, vasculitis, and idiopathic.

Table 31.1

Venous	Arterial	Diabetic
Single, large ulcer with **sloping edges** on medial retromalleolar (or **gaiter**) region, with unhealthy granulation tissue at base	Painful ulcers between toes or on pressure bearing areas. Regular **punched out edges**, with sloughy or necrotic base. Cold, pale foot, with signs of chronic ischaemia present	Ulcer punched out of surrounding callous, on pressure-bearing area of foot. Toes are clawed, with warm skin and **glove and stocking** sensory loss

c. LYMPHATIC DISORDERS

What are the signs of lymphoedema?

Lymphoedema is oedema arising principally from a failure of lymph drainage, resulting in a swollen limb with non-pitting oedema.
Skin changes are also apparent, giving a **cobblestone appearance**.
Kaposi–Stemmer sign is present.

What are the causes of unilateral lymphoedema?

Pelvic tumour
Malignant lymphatic invasion
Idiopathic
Lymphatic surgery
Radiotherapy
Lymphatic filariasis.

How would you treat lymphoedema?

Conservative: multilayer bandaging, exercise, and manual lymph drainage (massage).
Watch for signs of infection and treat early (predisposition to cellulitis).
Consider prophylactic antibiotics if infection becomes recurrent.
Surgical: In severe disability only; subcutaneous tissue is removed and skin graft used to cover defect.

CHAPTER 32: BENIGN BREAST DISEASE

What is the axiom of breast disease?
'No woman should remain with a lump in her breast.'

What is mastalgia?
Breast pain. May be **cyclical** or **non-cyclical**.

What is the significance of mastalgia?
The majority of breast pain (>90%) is attributed to the breasts' normal cyclical changes under hormonal effects, especially in the pre-menstrual period.

What is cyclical mastalgia?
Mastalgia occurring with menstruation.
If suspected, can be confirmed by asking the patient to keep a diary of when they have the pain in relation to their menstruation.
Cyclical pain does not require treatment in most cases and reassurance is sufficient.
In severe cases, primrose oil, danazol, and bromocriptine have been proven effective in symptom relief.

What can cause non-cyclical mastalgia?
Breast abscess (see Chapter 24). A very small proportion of patients presenting with breast pain may have underlying breast malignancy and although this is rare, it needs to be excluded through triple assessment.

What is the triple assessment?
1. Clinical examination
2. Imaging: USS/mammogram
3. Fine needle aspiration cytology (FNAC).

Who gets triple assessment?
All women presenting with a breast lump!

What form of imaging is available?

Mammography: most common form of imaging used to assess the breast and is routinely used for **cancer screening**. Two views are usually obtained: **oblique** and **craniocaudal**. False negative rate = 10%.
USS: used in younger patients (<35 years old) because radiodensity of the breasts is higher and lumps are not easily detectable with mammography. Used instead of or in conjunction with mammography.

What is ANDI?

ANDI stands for Abnormalities of the Normal Development and Involution of the breast ie referring to all benign breast disease.

What abnormalities of breast development are there?

Accessory nipples/breasts
Asymmetry: some degree of asymmetry is normal (left is usually larger)
Juvenile hypertrophy: affecting either one or, more commonly, both breasts
Fibroadenomas.

What is the milk line?

The milk line runs from the axilla down to the groin bilaterally and accessory nipples/breasts may appear anywhere along this line. Accessory nipples/breasts are benign but patients often seek medical advice due to cosmetic reasons.

What is the most common reason for a 30-year-old presenting with a breast lump?

Fibroadenomas: benign breast lumps caused by overgrowth of normal breast tissue, arising from a single breast lobule. Most commonly seen in young women 20–35 years old and make up 20% of all breast lumps.

How does a fibroadenoma present?	As a single, well demarcated breast lump which is firm in nature and mobile (Syn. **breast mouse**).
How is it differentiated from breast carcinoma?	Triple assessment.
What is its cancer risk?	Fibroadenomas are not a pre-malignant condition nor are patients at an increased risk of developing breast cancer later on.
What is the most common reason for a 50-year-old presenting with a breast lump?	**Breast cysts:** benign lumps that arise from a variation of normal lobular change and make up 15% of all breast lumps seen. Most commonly affect postmenopausal women; may be single or multiple.
How do breast cysts present?	As firm, discrete, mobile lumps which may or may not feel fluctuant on examination. They may be painful.
How are they managed?	Triple assessment! FNAC can be therapeutic as well as diagnostic but cysts rarely need treatment other than patient reassurance.
Are breast cysts malignant?	May be perceived as a malignant lump by the patient but are **benign**. Simple cysts disappear on aspiration. Suspicious signs include: 1. Aspirating blood-stained fluid 2. Positive cytology from the aspirate 3. Recurrent persistent cysts 4. Abnormal imaging. Malignancy must be ruled out.
What types of nipple discharge are there?	**Milky:** physiological, lactation **Green/yellow:** mastitis, duct ectasia **Bloody:** duct papillomas, ductal carcinoma *in situ*, duct ectasia, malignancy.

What is duct ectasia?

Abnormal dilation of the peri-areolar ducts.

Green/cream secretions may collect in these, provoking chronic inflammation and fibrosis of the ducts. Result: nipple discharge, nipple retraction, and predisposition to breast abscesses. Bilateral condition.

What is gynaecomastia?

Enlargement of the breast tissue in males.

What are the causes?

Drugs (digoxin, cimetidine, diamorphine, spironolactone, vincristine, oestrogens)
Hormones (cortisol [Cushing's], prolactin [prolactinoma], growth hormone [puberty, acromegaly], thyroid hormone [hyperthyroidism])
Teratoma
Cannabis
Liver failure (cirrhosis, primary biliary cirrhosis, alcoholism)
Renal failure.

For an algorithm on management of a breast lump, and the management of breast cancer, see Chapter 43.

CHAPTER 33: ENDOCRINE DISORDERS

a. THYROID

APPLIED ANATOMY

What are the parts of the gland?	Two lobes joined in the midline by the thyroid isthmus.
Where does it lie?	In front of the 2nd, 3rd and 4th tracheal rings.
What is its blood supply?	Superior and inferior thyroid aa. from the external carotid a. and thyrocervical trunk respectively.
What two nerves must be preserved during thyroidectomy?	The recurrent laryngeal and superior laryngeal nn.
Where does the recurrent laryngeal nerve run?	Lateral to the gland on both sides in the tracheo-oesophageal groove.
What is its relationship to the inferior thyroid artery?	Usually *behind* the artery on the left, but has a 50% chance of being either in front of or behind the artery on the right.
How are these two nerves preserved during thyroidectomy?	By clamping the superior thyroid a. at the superior thyroid pole (where it enters), hence preserving the superior laryngeal n.; and clamping the inferior thyroid a. *lateral* to the inferior pole (where it enters), hence preserving the recurrent laryngeal n.

CLINICAL CONSIDERATIONS

What is a goitre?	An enlargement of the thyroid gland.
How can goitre be classified?	**Non-toxic (simple) goitre:** • Diffuse hyperplastic • Nodular

Toxic goitre:
- Diffuse (**Graves' disease**)
- Multinodular.

Neoplastic goitre:
- Benign:
  - Follicular adenoma
- Malignant:
  - Papillary
  - Follicular
  - Medullary
  - Anaplastic
  - Lymphoma.

Thyroiditis:
- Autoimmune (**Hashimoto's disease**)
- Granulomatous (subacute; **De Quervain's**)
- Benign inflammatory (**Riedel's**)
- Acute (bacterial; **rare**).

What clinical states of thyroid function do you know of?

$\downarrow$ Function = hypothyroid
Normal function = euthyroid
$\uparrow$ Function = hyperthyroid

What are the thyroid hormones and which one is the active form?

Thyroxine (T_4) and tri-iodothyronine (T_3).
T_3 is the active form.
Thyroid hormone production is regulated by thyroid stimulating hormone (TSH), produced by the anterior pituitary gland.

What are the indications for thyroid surgery?

The 4 Cs:
Cosmesis (the cosmetic effect of neck swelling)
Compression (may cause respiratory distress or dysphagia by compressing trachea and oesophagus respectively)
Control (of toxic symptoms in hyperthyroidism)
Carcinoma.

NON-TOXIC (SIMPLE) GOITRE

What causes simple goitre?

1. Iodine deficiency (<100 μg/day): iodinated salt has revolutionised this.
2. Defects in thyroid hormone synthesis
   a. Enzyme deficiency (various enzymes along the thyroid hormone synthesis pathway may be deficient 2ry to genetic predisposition)
   b. Goitrogens (inhibit organic binding of iodine)
      i. Vegetables such as cabbage, cassava and rape
      ii. Antithyroid drugs.

What is the connection between hyperplastic and nodular goitre?

Simple hyperplastic may give rise to nodular through a cycle of degeneration and regeneration of thyroid follicles. Both, however, are **euthyroid**.

How is simple goitre managed?

Prevention is the key (eg iodinated salt), but in established cases, the following are available:
Conservative: for **early hyperplastic goitre** only; give thyroxine, which may cause regression.
Surgical: for **late hyperplastic** and **nodular goitre** (irreversible); surgery for cosmesis or compression.

HYPERTHYROIDISM

What are the causes?

Graves' disease and toxic multinodular goitre.

What is Graves' disease?

An autoimmune disease, affecting mainly young women (F:M = 6:1), associated with hyperthyroidism and eye symptoms.

Symptoms are due to the production of **thyroid stimulating antibodies** (TsAb) which act at and sensitise thyroid TSH receptors. The thyroid gland becomes uniformly **hyperplastic** and **hypertrophied**.

What is toxic multinodular goitre?

One which usually arises from a long-standing simple nodular goitre, affecting the middle-aged and elderly (M=F). Patients become hyperthyroid, but there is no autoimmune process, and eye symptoms are **absent**. Palpable nodules may either be **solitary** or **multiple**.

What are the symptoms of hyperthyroidism?

There may be a **discrete neck swelling**, but the patient may also complain of the following:
General: sweating, heat intolerance, weight loss
Cardiovascular: palpitations, chest pain
Neurological: tremor, anxiety, mood swings
Gastrointestinal: hyperdefecation or diarrhoea
Gynaecological: menstrual irregularities.

What are the signs in hyperthyroidism?

General: Anxious, fidgety patient; weight loss.
Hands (7 signs):
1. Sweating
2. Fine, resting tremor
3. Palmar erythema
4. Clubbing (thyroid acropathy; *Graves' only*)
5. Onycholysis (nail destruction; *Graves' only*)
6. Vitiligo (*Graves' only*)
7. Pulse: tachycardia and arrhythmias.

Eyes *(7 signs; Graves' only):*

1. Loss of outer 1/3 of eyebrow
2. Lid retraction ($\uparrow$ sympathetic response)
3. Lid lag (CN III palsy)
4. Ophthalmoplegia (CN III, IV & VI palsies)
5. Chemosis
6. Proptosis
7. Exophthalmos.

Neck:

Graves' disease: diffuse, symmetrically enlarged gland with audible bruit (due to hypervascularity).

Toxic multinodular goitre: solitary or multiple palpable nodules; gland may be irregular.

NB Look for scar of previous thyroid surgery.

Other: pretibial myxoedema; proximal myopathy; $\uparrow$ reflexes; hepatomegaly (rare).

What is the difference between proptosis and exophthalmos?

Proptosis: bulging of the eyeball past the supraorbital ridge, as seen from above and behind.

Exophthalmos: the limbus (the region of cornea surrounding the iris) can be seen both above and below the iris (usually only seen below).

What are the investigations?

Blood investigations:

Thyroid function tests (TFTs): $\uparrow T_3/T_4$; $\downarrow$TSH.

Hypocholesterolaemia.

Antibody studies can also be done in Graves' disease.

Imaging:

USS: especially if multinodular; differentiates between solid nodules and cysts.

Scintigraphy: ^{123}I is injected and taken up by thyroid gland. ↑ diffuse uptake in Graves' disease; ↑ discrete uptake in toxic multinodular goitre ('**hot spots**')

What is the management?

Conservative:
1. Antithyroid drugs: carbimazole or propylthiouracil
2. β-blockers for cardiac and sympathetic symptoms.

Irradiation: radioactive iodine can be used to ablate gland; pt. swallows ^{123}I which is taken up by gland. External beam is then focused on thyroid gland. Side-effects are hypothyroidism, cancer risk, and infertility. Reserved for **older patients** (>25 years). *Rarely used in toxic multinodular goitre.*

Surgical: for **control**, especially when other modalities have failed, or in pregnancy. Popular in **young patients**. A **subtotal thyroidectomy** is performed (some thyroid tissue is left behind). Pt. *must* be covered with carbimazole and β-blockers before surgery to prevent **thyroid storm**.

What is a thyroid storm?

An **acute exacerbation** of hyperthyroidism. May occur during handling of the thyroid at surgery: excessive amounts of thyroid hormone may be released into the circulation causing massive sympathetic response and cardiovascular compromise. Rx: hydrocortisone, β-blockers, carbimazole, Lugol's iodine, and digoxin (for atrial fibrillation).

| What other complications of thyroidectomy do you know? | **Early:**
Haemorrhage (an emergency; evacuate on ward!)
Recurrent laryngeal nerve damage
Respiratory compromise (usually 2ry to laryngeal oedema).
Late:
Hypothyroidism
Hypocalcaemia (from inadvertent damage or removal of parathyroids)
Wound complications (infection, keloid). |
| **What *must* be at the bedside of a patient who has had a thyroidectomy?** | A clip remover in case of an acute bleed. |

HYPOTHYROIDISM

| What are its causes? | 1. Autoimmune (Hashimoto's disease)
2. Iodine deficiency
3. Post-irradiation
4. Tumour infiltration
5. Anti-thyroid drug therapy
6. Hypopituitarism (↓thyrotropin releasing hormone [TRH] which leads to ↓TSH release from the anterior pituitary). |
| **What are the symptoms of hypothyroidism?** | Patient may have a discrete neck swelling, but may also complain of the following:
General: cold intolerance; change in voice/hoarseness; weight gain; dry skin with pruritis; hair loss
Neurological: depression, lethargy, psychosis (**myxoedema madness**)
Gastrointestinal: constipation
Gynaecological: menstrual irregularities.
NB Pt. may also present in **hypothyroid coma**. |

What are the signs of hypothyroidism?	**General:** lethargic, overweight, hair loss **Hands:** Thick, dry, doughy skin; bradycardia **Other:** ↓ reflexes.
What are the investigations?	**Blood investigations:** Thyroid function tests (TFTs): ↑TSH; ↓T_3/T_4. Hypercholesterolaemia.
What is the management?	Oral thyroxine.
What is infantile hypo-thyroidism called?	Cretinism. Goitre results in **star-gazing sign** (the enlarged goitre causes hyperextension of the neck). Usually caused by maternal use of anti-thyroid drugs which cross the placenta (propylthiouracil).

THYROIDITIS

What is Hashimoto's disease?	An autoimmune disease causing **lymphocytic infiltration** of the thyroid gland with resulting hypothyroidism. The main antibody formed is **antithyroglobulin**. F>M (95%). Thyroid becomes **firm and rubbery**. Rx: thyroxine.
What is De Quervain's thyroiditis?	A subacute, **viral** thyroiditis which causes a swollen, tender thyroid which undergoes **granulomatous change**. Self-resolving. Rx: NSAIDs +/− steroids.
What is Riedel's thyroiditis?	A benign inflammatory thyroid enlargement. The thyroid undergoes **fibrotic change** which may spread to surrounding tissues. The thyroid becomes **wooden** in texture and may be difficult to differentiate from carcinoma. Rx: none.

What is acute thyroiditis?	A bacterial infection of the thyroid gland, usually *Streptococcus* or *Staphylococcus*. Bacteria has usually seeded up a thyroglossal fistula (see below). Rx: antibiotics based on cultures.

OTHER THYROID CONDITIONS

What is a thyroglossal duct?	A patent tract occurring along the line of descent of the thyroid gland during its embryonic development. It runs from the base of the tongue (the original site of the primitive thyroid gland) to the gland itself. It is usually tethered by the middle third of the **hyoid bone**.
What is a thyroglossal cyst?	A **midline neck swelling** representing a cystic swelling of an otherwise non-patent thyroglossal tract.
How can it classically be differentiated from other midline neck swellings?	By protrusion of the tongue. Because it is tethered by the thyroglossal tract, tongue protrusion causes it to move upwards.
What is the main complication?	Thyroglossal **fistula** formation from I and D of a cyst which has become infected.

For management of thyroid carcinoma and the solitary thyroid nodule, see Chapter 48.

b. PARATHYROID

APPLIED ANATOMY

How many parathyroid glands?	4 in all.

Where do they lie?	Usually behind the superior and inferior poles of the thyroid gland. The position of the two superior ones is more constant, whilst the inferior ones may be quite variable in position (eg in thyroid substance, lower neck and mediastinum).
Where do the parathyroids originate from?	**Superior glands:** 4th pharyngeal pouch **Inferior glands:** 3rd pharyngeal pouch (same as the thymus which displaces them caudally, accounting for their sometimes variable positions).
How is serum calcium regulated?	See Figure 33.1.

Figure 33.1 Regulation of serum calcium

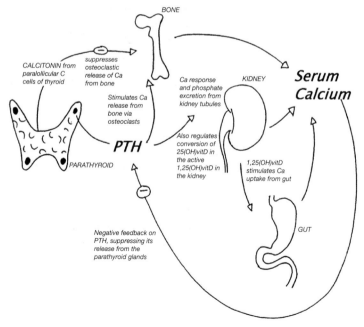

How can hyperparathyroidism be classified?	As 1ry, 2ry or 3ry: **1ry:** from parathyroid hyperplasia (1–4 glands may be affected; 10%), adenoma (85%), or carcinoma (1%). **2ry:** low serum Ca^{2+}, such as in **renal failure** or **gut malabsorption**, causes a rise in PTH levels. Serum Ca^{2+} levels are normal or low. **3ry:** long-standing 2ry hyperparathyroidism, such as in chronic renal failure, causes parathyroid hyperplasia. Serum Ca^{2+} levels are high.
How does the patient present?	With symptoms of hypercalcaemia: *mnemonic* **'Bones, moans, stones and abdominal groans'** **Bones:** bone pain, osteoclastomas **Moans:** depression and lethargy **Stones:** renal calculi **Abdominal groans:** PUD, constipation, pancreatitis. NB Most patients are **asymptomatic** and hyperparathyroidism is usually an **incidental finding** in the blood results.
What are the clinical findings?	Usually very little. There may be hypertension.
What are the investigations?	**Blood investigations:** ↑PTH, ↑Ca^{2+} (except in 2ry), ↓PO_4 **Imaging:** **X-ray:** 1. Subperiosteal bone resorption (seen at phalanges; **pathognomonic**)

2. **Pepper-pot skull** (skull film punctuated with circular areas of radiolucency, like a pepper pot; due to bone resorption in an attempt to $\uparrow$Ca^{2+} levels).
CT scan: gives anatomical detail of glands, especially if in aberrant locations.
Technetium-thallium subtraction scan also useful.

What are the differentials of hypercalcaemia?

mnemonic: **HI CALCIUM Produces Stones**
Hyperparathyroidism(1ry, 2ry or 3ry)/
Hypocalciuric hypercalcaemia (familial)
Iatrogenic: thiazide diuretics
Calcium and vitamins A & D excess
Addison's disease/**A**cromegaly
Lung (pulmonary) TB
Carcinoma (breast, prostate, lung, kidney, thyroid)
Immobility
Unrelated: ectopic PTH production (lung, kidney, ovary carcinoma)
Multiple myeloma/**M**ilk-alkali syndrome (rare)
Paget's disease of bone
Sarcoidosis ($\uparrow$ vitamin D action)

What is the management?

Definitive treatment depends on the type of hyperparathyroidism.
1ry: surgery (depends on pathology):
Hyperplasia: remove all 4 glands, and replace 30 mg of parathyroid tissue in forearm (maintains parathyroid function, and easily removed if PTH rises again).
Adenoma: remove affected gland and biopsy other 3.
Carcinoma: remove affected gland and ipsilateral thyroid lobe and lymph nodes.

2ry: parathyroids are not the problem here. Renal failure is. Correct Ca^{2+} and PO_4 levels. Pt. needs renal transplant.

3ry: as with 2ry, but parathyroid hyperplasia has now occurred. Correct Ca^{2+} and PO_4 levels, perform renal transplant, and finally excise all 4 parathyroids and implant 30 mg of tissue in forearm.

In all **acute** cases, IV fluids and diuretics (*not* thiazides) should be administered pre-op to counteract **dehydration**.

What must be ruled out in 1ry hyperparathyroidism due to hyperplasia?	MEN syndrome (see below).

HYPOPARATHYROIDISM

What is the most common cause?	Surgical removal, either with intention or inadvertently, following thyroidectomy, parathyroidectomy or radical neck surgery.
What are the symptoms?	Those of **hypocalcaemia**: parasthaesia (at digits and circumorally), cramps, psychosis. Pt. May also present **fitting**.
What are the signs?	***Hands:*** paraesthesia; **Trousseau's sign** (spasm/clawing of the fingers when BP cuff is inflated around arm for 3 minutes). ***Face:*** circumoral paraesthesia; **Chvostek's sign** (twitching of facial muscles when tapping on facial nerve).

What are the other causes of hypocalcaemia?	Acute pancreatitis (acidosis and fat necrosis)
	Massive transfusion (contained **citrate** is a Ca^{2+} chelating agent)
	Vitamin D deficiency ($\downarrow$ gut absorption and $\uparrow$ renal excretion of Ca^{2+})
	Chronic renal failure ($\downarrow$ activation of vitamin D 2ry to $\downarrow$ 1-α hydroxylase production)
What are the investigations?	**Blood investigations:** $\downarrow Ca^{2+}$, $\uparrow PO_4$
	Imaging: CT scan or technetium-thallium scan of neck can be done if cause is thought to be inadvertent surgical removal.
What is the management?	1. IV calcium gluconate (acutely)
	2. Oral vitamin D preparations
	3. Oral calcium preparations.

c. ADRENAL

APPLIED ANATOMY

What does the adrenal gland produce?	Depends on the area. It comprises an outer **cortex** and an inner **medulla**. The **cortex** has 3 zones:
	mnemonic: from outside in, **GFR** (remembered by the fact that the adrenal sits atop the kidney where the glomerular filtration rate, or GFR, is important!):
	zona Glomerulosa (outer): mineralocorticoids
	zona Fasciculata (middle): glucocorticoids and androgens
	zona Reticulata (inner): oestrogens.
	The **medulla** produces the catecholamines epinephrine (adrenaline; 80%) and norepinephrine (noradrenaline; 10%).

What is the main glucocorticoid?	Cortisol.
How is it controlled?	Via a feedback loop: **corticotropin releasing hormone** (**CRH**) from the anterior hypothalamus stimulates **adrenocorticotrophic hormone** (**ACTH**) release from the anterior pituitary, which in turn stimulates cortisol release from the adrenal gland. Cortisol negatively feeds back to CRH and ACTH.
What is the main mineralocorticoid?	Aldosterone.
How is it controlled?	By the **renin-angiotensin-aldosterone axis**. Fall in BP is sensed as ↓ renal perfusion by the kidney which causes renin release from its juxtoglomerular apparatus. This stimulates angiotensin (and its active metabolite angiotensin II) production in the lung, which has a direct vasoconstrictive effect and causes aldosterone release from the adrenal gland. Aldosterone causes salt retention by acting on the collecting ducts of the kidney.

CUSHING'S SYNDROME

What is Cushing's syndrome?	A clinical syndrome of glucocorticoid excess.
What are the causes?	Iatrogenic (excess steroid use) Pituitary adenoma (excess ACTH) Corticoadrenal adenoma/carcinoma (excess cortisol) ACTH-producing tumours (eg oat-cell lung CA; ACTH produced is *much* higher than that produced in pituitary adenoma).

What is Cushing's syndrome secondary to pituitary adenoma also known as?	Cushing's *disease*.
What are the clinical features?	*General:* thin limbs (from proximal muscle wasting) with **truncal obesity** (classically: 'like a lemon on match-sticks'); fat deposits at the back of the neck (**buffalo hump**). *Face:* fat redistribution and around the face (**moon face**); hair loss. *Skin:* acne, ecchymoses, striae and poorly healing wounds (from thin, fragile skin). *Neurological:* depression; proximal myopathy.
What do they develop?	Diabetes mellitus (cortisol is **glucogenic**) and hypertension.
What are the investigations?	**Blood investigations:** 1. U+Es: may be deranged 2. Random blood sugar: usually ↑ 3. Serum cortisol (normally high in am, low in pm [**circadian rhythm**]): persistently raised (loss of circadian rhythm) 4. Serum ACTH: raised in Cushing's disease and ACTH-producing tumours. **Urine:** A 24-hour urine test for **free cortisol** and **17-hydroxycorticosterone** (17-OHCS; a breakdown product of cortisol) should also be done. **Special tests:** Dexamethasone suppression test **Imaging:** 1. Pituitary CT scan 2. Adrenal CT scan 3. CXR for ACTH-producing oat-cell lung CA.

What is dexamethasone?

A synthetic glucocorticoid. It is more potent than cortisol.

What is the dexamethasone suppression test?

A test for Cushing's syndrome. There is a low-dose and a high-dose test. Start with the low dose.

Low-dose: 2 mg dex given @ midnight and either serum or urine cortisol is checked in the morning:

→ **Low cortisol:** no Cushing's syndrome (as there is a normal negative feedback response on ACTH production).

→ **High cortisol:** Cushing's syndrome present (no negative feedback as either too much ACTH or cortisol being produced).

To determine the cause of Cushing's syndrome, perform high-dose test:

High-dose: 4 mg dex given and test repeated:

→ **Low cortisol:** no Cushing's syndrome, or Cushing's syndrome 2ry to Cushing's disease (pituitary cause; hi-dose dex *overrides* excess ACTH production by pituitary, causing negative feedback)

→ **High cortisol:** Cushing's syndrome 2ry to either ectopic ACTH-producing tumour (ACTH level still too high to be overridden) or adrenal tumour (too much cortisol to suppress)

Imaging above to determine cause further.

Can you summarise the above?

See Table 33.1.

Table 33.1

Cause of Cushing's syndrome	Cortisol level (serum/urine)	ACTH level	Dexamethasone suppression test
Normal patients	Normal	Normal	Low: suppression High: suppression
Pituitary adenoma (Cushing's disease)	High	High	Low: no suppression High: suppression
Adrenal tumour	High	Low	Low: no suppression High: no suppression
Ectopic ACTH-producing tumour	High	High	Low: no suppression High: no suppression

What is the management?

Conservative: reserved for 2 cases:
1. Severe cortisol excess; Rx: **metyrapone** (blocks cortisol synthesis)
2. Inoperable adrenal carcinoma; Rx: **mitotane** (selectively kills cortisol-producing cells).

Otherwise, treatment is **surgical**:
Pituitary adenoma: trans-sphenoidal excision of adenoma (alternatively external-beam irradiation may be used)
Adrenal adenoma: adrenalectomy
Adrenal carcinoma: excision
Ectopic ACTH-producing tumour: excision (where feasible).

What is Nelson's syndrome?

A syndrome of **pituitary enlargement** following bilateral adrenalectomy (20% of cases; caused by removal of cortisol and hence source of negative feedback on pituitary). Symptoms include:
• Hyperpigmentation ($\uparrow$ pituitary pro-opiomelanocortin [POMC] production which $\uparrow$ melanin production)

- Headaches (↑ intracranial pressure)
- Visual field defects (optic nerve compression).

CONN'S SYNDROME

What is Conn's syndrome?	A clinical syndrome of hyperaldosteronism.
What are the causes?	Corticoadrenal adenoma (most common) Corticoadrenal hyperplasia Corticoadrenal carcinoma.
What are the two classic signs of Conn's syndrome?	**Hypertension** and **hypokalaemia**.
Can you explain this?	**Hypertension:** aldosterone acts on renal collecting ducts, causing salt retention. This in turn ↑ intravascular compartment and hence BP. **Hypokalaemia:** the receptors aldosterone acts on cause simultaneous Na^+ retention and K^+ excretion.
How does the patient present?	Fatigue, muscle weakness, thirst, polyuria and nocturia. HTN is found on examination.
What are the investigations?	**Blood investigations:** U+Es for ↑Na^+, ↓K^+ **Special tests:** 1. **Saline infusion test**: infusion will ↓ aldosterone in normal patients (negative feedback mechanism); remains high in Conn's syndrome 2. **Captopril test:** ↓ aldosterone levels in normal patients by causing ↓ in the stimulatory angiotensin II; no effect in Conn's syndrome.

Imaging:
1. CT scan
2. Cholesterol scanning (cholesterol needed in mineralo- and glucocorticoid synthesis; high uptake in Conn's syndrome).

What is the treatment?

Depends on the pathology:
Adenoma: adrenalectomy
Hyperplasia: if unilateral, adrenalectomy; if bilateral, give **spironolactone** (K^+-sparing diuretic) only
Carcinoma: adrenalectomy (if feasible).
NB All patients must be covered with spironolactone pre-operatively.

ADDISON'S DISEASE

What is Addison's disease?

A clinical syndrome of adrenocortical insufficiency. Both mineralo- and glucocorticoids are undersecreted.

What are the causes?

Autoimmune (most common; 60%).
Iatrogenic (bilateral adrenalectomy)
Corticoadrenal carcinoma
Sudden withdrawal of steroid therapy
Infection (classically TB).

What are the classic signs?

Hypotension and **hyperkalaemia** (due to hypoaldosteronism, the opposite of Conn's syndrome).

How does the patient present?

Hyperpigmentation (2ry to no negative feedback on pituitary causing ↑ POMC production [as in Nelson's syndrome]); postural hypotension. Pt. may present with an **Addisonian crisis**.

What is an Addisonian crisis?	Acute adrenal insufficiency, usually in the face of a stressor such as surgery or trauma. The normal rise in **glucocorticoids** in response to stress is impaired. Pt. becomes hypotensive with nausea, vomiting, diarrhoea and abdominal pain. May go into shock. **Rx:** IV fluids, IV hydrocortisone and oral fludrocortisone (a mineralocorticoid).
What are the investigations?	**Blood investigations:** U+Es for ↓Na$^+$, ↑K$^+$ **Special tests: Short Synacthen test,** whereby Synacthen, a synthetic ACTH analogue, is administered. It causes an ↑ in cortisol in normal patients, but has no effect in Addison's disease.
What is Waterhouse–Friderichsen syndrome?	A syndrome of adrenocortical haemorrhage and insufficiency caused by meningococcal septicaemia.

PHAEOCHROMOCYTOMA

What is phaeochromocytoma?	An adrenal medulla tumour of the **chromaffin cells** which produces excess catecholamines.
Which catecholamine is most produced?	Norepinephrine > epinephrine.
Who gets it?	Anyone of any age, but most common in 40–60 year olds.
What is the classic triad of symptoms?	1. Palpitations 2. Headache 3. Periodic excessive sweating. Pt. may also c/o anxiety, flushing, weight loss and angina, and may occasionally present as a stroke.

What is the classic presentation of bladder phaeochromocytoma?	The above triad on urination.
What is found on examination?	Mainly sweating, arrhythmias and **hypertension**.
What is the rule of 10s of phaeochromocytoma?	**The rule of 10s is as follows:** 1. 10% malignant 2. 10% bilateral 3. 10% in children 4. 10% multiple tumours 5. 10% extra-adrenal (thorax, neck, bladder, kidney, scrotum) 6. 10% familial (von Hippel–Lindau syndrome, MEN I & II).
What are the investigations?	**Blood investigations:** ↑ Random blood sugar (catecholamines are glucogenic) Serum epinephrine and norepinephrine levels **Special tests:** 24-hour urinary **vanillylmandelic acid** (**VMA**) levels (breakdown product of catecholamines); **gold standard test**. **Imaging:** 1. CT scan or MRI for localisation 2. ^{131}I-MIBG (methyliodobenzylguanidine) scan (a radioiodine-labelled catecholamine analogue which is taken up by the tumour) 3. IVC venous sampling if all else fails (catecholamine levels help localise tumour).
What is the treatment?	**Conservative:** should start *at diagnosis* and continue right up to the pre-operative period; administer α-**blockers** (prazosin or phenoxybenzamine).

Surgical: Excision of tumour with early ligation of venous drainage to avoid **hypertensive crisis** during handling.

How is a hypertensive crisis managed?

With **nitroprusside**.

What is von Hippel–Lindau syndrome?

See p. 25.

d. MULTIPLE ENDOCRINE NEOPLASIA (MEN) SYNDROME

What is MEN syndrome?

An autosomal dominant predisposition to developing multiple endocrine tumours.

What types do you know of?

3 types:
MEN I (Wermer's syndrome)
Parathyroid hyperplasia
Pancreatic islet cell tumour:
    Zollinger–Ellison syndrome (50%)
    Insulinoma (20%)
Pituitary tumours
mnemonic: type 1 = **p**rimary = pathology beginning with **P**.
MEN IIA (Sipple's syndrome)
Medullary thyroid carcinoma
Phaeochromocytoma
Hyperparathyroidism (parathyroid hyperplasia)
mnemonic: type 2 = **s**econdary = **S**ipple's; pts. with MEN type **2**a drive @ **2** mph (**MPH**).
MEN IIB
Medullary thyroid carcinoma
Mucosal neuromas
Phaeochromocytoma
Marfanoid body habitus
mnemonic: pts. with MEN type 2b enjoy **M**&**M**s in the afternoon (**PM**)

CHAPTER 34: UROLOGICAL DISEASE

a. URINARY TRACT INFECTIONS (UTIS)

What types do you know of?	Lower UTI and upper UTI (pyelonephritis).
Who are more prone to them?	Women due to the short length of the female urethra; UTI in males is *rare*.
What are the causative organisms?	*E. coli* (80%) *Staphylococcus saprophyticus* (5–15%) *Ureaplasma urealyticum* STDs: *Chlamydia trachomatis* *Neisseria gonnorhoeae* (rarely).
What increases the likelihood of a male contracting a lower UTI?	1. Unprotected anal intercourse 2. Lack of circumcision 3. Intercourse with a female whose vagina is colonised by uropathogens 4. Anatomical abnormality (eg posterior urethral valves).
How does lower UTI present?	Pyuria, dysuria, urgency and frequency.
What are the investigations?	1. Urine dipstick will show leucocytes $+/-$ blood; if *Ureaplasma* is present, nitrites will be positive. 2. MSU for M/C/S 3. Renal tract imaging (1st episode in men; recurrent UTI in women).
What is considered significant on MSU for a UTI?	Quantitative culture yield of $> 10^5$ bacteria/ml.
What is the treatment?	**Education (females):** wipe from front to back after defecation; don't soak in the bath for long periods; wear cotton underwear instead of synthetic fabrics.

Medical: trimethoprim/
suxamethonium (TMP/SMX) or
fluoroquinolones (eg ciprofloxacin) for
3 days; use for 7 days if patient is
diabetic, symptomatic for >7 days,
has been having recurrent UTIs, is
>65 years old, or is using a
contraceptive diaphragm.

**How else can lower UTI
present in men?**

As epididymo-orchitis (see Chapter
27) or prostatitis (see later).

**How does pyelonephritis
present?**

Fever, flank pain, and lower UTI
symptoms. There is renal angle
tenderness on percussion on the
renal angle. Patient may have
nausea, vomiting, and rigors.

What is the treatment?

Mild/moderate: 10–14 day course
of oral TMP/SMX or fluoroquinolones
Severe: IV fluoroquinolones or
aminoglycosides (eg gentamicin).

**What is the next step if
there is no resolution after
48 hours?**

1. Change antibiotic to match
   urinary culture result
2. Imaging (KUB USS, IVU, spiral CT
   scan) to r/o intrarenal or
   perinephric abscess or calculi
3. Treat underlying cause, if any.

b. RENAL CALCULI

APPLIED ANATOMY

**What are the parts of the
urinary tract?**

See Figure 34.1.

**What are the narrowest
points?**

3 points to remember:
1. Pelvi-ureteric junction
2. Point at which the ureter crosses
   the pelvic brim
3. Vesico-ureteric junction.

Figure 34.1 The urinary tract

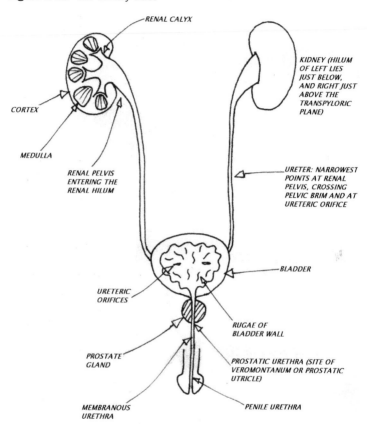

What is the clinical significance of this?	They represent the most common points that calculi can get lodged and potentially cause urinary retention.
What is the diameter of the ureter?	Approximately 3 mm.
So why is *this* important to know?	Stones bigger than 3 mm in diameter will have a greater propensity to lodge (they can be measured on X-ray).

What prevents reflux of urine back into the ureters from the bladder?

The oblique angle at which the ureters enter the bladder at its trigone. This acts as a valve mechanism.

What is the presence of renal calculi also known as?

Nephrolithiasis.

What types of stones do you know of?

1. **Calcium stones (75%):** 3 types:
   a. Oxalate
   b. Phosphate
   c. Urate.
   Can be caused by and are a cause of hypercalcaemia (see Chapter 4). Ca oxalate stones also caused by $\uparrow$ ingestion of oxalate-containing compounds (eg rhubarb, tea).
2. **Struvite stones (15%):** made up magnesium ammonium phosphate ($MgNH_4PO_4$). Caused by urea-splitting organisms (*Proteus*, *Pseudomonas*, *Klebsiella*). Released ammonium binds Mg and PO_4.
3. **Uric acid stones (6%):** caused by:
   a. $\uparrow$ Purine uptake (eg meat, legumes)
   b. Gout
   c. $\uparrow$ Cell turnover (eg malignancy).
4. **Cystine stones (2%):** caused by cystinuria, an abnormality in uptake of cystine, amongst other amino acids, from the urine.
The causes of all of the above stones should be determined during the history.

What else should you ask?

1. Previous history of stones and intervention taken if any (may have had stones or an entire kidney removed in the past)

2. Factors precipitating symptoms, such as dehydration or following a beer binge (*classic presentation;* beer is a diuretic, causing excessive urination and contraction of the kidney around its contained stone).

Who gets stones?

M:F = 3:1; more common in 3rd and 4th decade

How do they present?

Depends on where they are in the urinary tract:
Renal: dull, aching flank pain without radiation, especially if stone is at **pelvi-ureteric junction**.
Ureteric: pt. experiences **renal colic** (better referred to as **ureteric colic**): wave-like spasms of pain, classically radiating from loin to groin.
Vesico-ureteric junction: iliac fossa pain with irritative symptoms (frequency and dysuria).
Bladder: may be asymptomatic or cause suprapubic pain and irritative symptoms.

What are the main differentials for ureteric colic?

In the RIF: **appendicitis**.
In females: **gynaecological emergencies** (L/RIF).

What is the main complication of renal calculi?

Urinary outflow obstruction and retention +/− superimposed proximal urinary tract infection.

Where are stones most likely to get lodged?

At the renal tract's narrowest points (see above).

When would a patient with nephrolithiasis need to be admitted?

In the following circumstances:
1. Uncontrolled pain with n/v
2. Urinary outflow obstruction
3. Proximal UTI (ie proximal to the stone).

What are the investigations?	**Blood investigations:**

What are the investigations?

Blood investigations:

1. **FBC**: anaemia 2ry to haematuria
2. **U+Es**: assess renal function, especially if retention is suspected; also, IVU is contraindicated in renal failure (Cr >2 g/dl) due to inability of kidney to excrete nephrotoxic dye
3. Bone profile: r/o hypercalcaemia
4. Uric acid: r/o gout.

Other: *urine dipstick is essential!* Dip urine to look for presence of UTI or blood. *If there is no blood on dipstick, re-think your diagnosis!* Besides leucocytes, pH > 7 suggests presence of urea-splitting organisms.

Imaging:

1. **KUB plain film:** look for presence of stones in the renal tract.
2. **IVU:** usually taken in conjunction with a KUB at 1, 5, 10 and 15 min post-injection of dye, until it fills both ureters; look for the following:
   a. Outline of the renal tract and stones if present
   b. Unilateral ureteral dilation (suggests a stone if not visible)
   c. Delayed nephrogram: nephrogram is an outline of the kidney with contrast; this is delayed in complete ureteric obstruction as dye cannot be excreted
   d. Hydronephrosis: blunting of the renal calyces due to urinary back-pressure
3. **KUB USS:** used in older patients when AAA (main differential in this age group) and malignancy should also be ruled out

4. **Spiral CT scan:** useful in further diagnosing difficult cases, or when IVU is contraindicated.

What percentage of kidney stones are visible on plain film?

90%.

What is the management?

1. IV analgesia and antiemetic
2. IV fluids
3. Strain urine for stones and send off for analysis.

Symptoms should settle down and stone should pass spontaneously with this. If complications occur (see above), then admit and treat accordingly.

Uncontrolled pain and obstruction: intervention to deal with stone; this is site dependent (see below).

Proximal UTI: antibiotics (gentamicin and ciprofloxacin).

What interventions are available to deal with stones?

Depends on the site:

Renal: percutaneous nephrolithotomy (PCNL): stones are removed percutaneously from the kidney.

Renal pelvis and proximal 1/3 of ureter:

Extracorporeal shockwave lithotripsy (ESWL): external shockwaves are used to shatter the stone while pt. sits in a tub of water; stone fragments are passed spontaneously.

Middle 1/3 of ureter: ureteric stenting: this widens the diameter of the ureter, facilitating spontaneous passage; if this fails, use ESWL or ureteroscopy (stone removed under direct vision by a ureteroscope passed up the ureter).

Lower 1/3 of ureter: ureteroscopy

Bladder: cystoscopy

c. PROSTATE

BENIGN PROSTATE HYPERPLASIA (BPH)

What is the prostate gland?	A male organ attached to bladder neck which forms the main bulk of ejaculate.
Can you describe it?	It is a chestnut shaped gland approximately 20 g in weight in the normal adult male.
What is its structure?	It is composed of **epithelial** and **stromal** elements. Epithelial cells form acinar glands whereas stroma forms collagen and smooth muscle fibres.
What are different zones of prostate?	Peripheral (70%), Central (25%), Transitional (5%). BPH mainly develops in the **transitional zone**.
What is BPH?	**Hyperplasia** resulting in increased number of cells both in epithelium and stroma. The proportion of hyperplasia affecting epithelial and stromal components varies in different patients.
What is its aetiology?	Unknown but it is considered to be an age related hormonal disease due to increased sensitisation of the prostate to **testosterone**.
What is the prevalence?	Most common benign tumour in males; prevalence is about 50% above 70 years. Its prevalence increases with age.

What are its main symptoms?

Symptoms are mainly divided into **obstructive** and **irritative**:

Obstructive (storage) symptoms:
- Poor stream
- Hesitancy
- Straining
- Terminal dribbling
- Urine retention.

Irritative (voiding) symptoms:
- Frequency
- Urgency
- Nocturia
- Urge incontinence
- Sense of incomplete evacuation.

How is the diagnosis of BPH made?

In addition to a relevant history (above), the following help:
1. Digital Rectal Examination (DRE)
2. Bladder USS, pre- and post-voiding to assess residual urine volume
3. Urine flow rates
4. Transrectal USS, to directly assess prostate (which lies against the lower rectal wall).

What are the classic findings of BPH on DRE?

An enlarged (>20 g), rubbery prostate with a clearly defined median sulcus and mobile overlying rectovesical fascia (of Denonvilliers).

What are the effects of BPH?

If left untreated, BPH can lead to:
1. Recurrent UTIs (2ry to urinary stasis)
2. Renal failure (post-renal, 2ry to bilateral ureteric outflow obstruction)
3. Urine retention (acute and chronic)
4. Bladder calculi (2ry to urinary stasis)
5. Detrusor failure (2ry to long-standing bladder enlargement).

What are the treatment options?

Watchful waiting: symptoms are mild
Medical: α-blockers and 5α-reductase inhibitors
Surgical: the following are indications for surgery:
- Where medical treatment has failed
- The presence of complications such as renal failure or calculi

The options are:
1. Transurethral resection of the prostate (TURP)
2. Transurethral laser-induced prostatectomy (TULIP)
3. Transurethral electrovaporisation of the prostate
4. Open prostatectomy (retropubic approach).

Long-term catheter: in patients not fit for surgery.

What are α-blockers?

α_1-adrenoreceptor antagonists.

What is the mechanism of actions of α-blockers?

The bladder neck and prostate contain α_1-adrenoreceptors. α-blockers act by blocking these receptors, causing relaxation of bladder neck and prostate, and hence, a better urinary flow.

What α-blockers do you know?

The α-blockers available are alfuzosin, terazosin and tamsulosin.

What is the mechanism of 5α-reductase inhibitors?

5α-reductase inhibitors block the conversion of testosterone to dihydrotestosterone, thus removing the stimulus for prostatic epithelial growth. The result is reduced prostatic size. They are generally used in combination with α-blockers.

What is an example of a 5α-reductase inhibitor?

Finasteride.

| **How is a TURP performed?** | A **resectoscope** (rigid lens-containing rod with an electrocautery loop at the end) is passed trans-urethrally (up the penis) and **prostatic chips** are cauterised away. A non-conducting irrigation fluid is used throughout the procedure. |

| **What fluids are used for TURP?** | Glycine-containing fluids. |

| **Why is normal saline not used for TURP?** | Because of its conducting abilities during resection. Glycine is non-conducting but it is absorbed because it is hypotonic. |

What are the complications of TURP?

The following are the main complications:
1. Retrograde ejaculation (80%)
2. Impotence (20%)
3. Stricture (1–2%)
4. Infection
5. Bleeding
6. TUR syndrome.

What is TUR syndrome?

Dilutional hyponitremia and **fluid overload** due to absorption of the hypotonic irrigation fluids (eg glycine-containing fluids) used during TURP into the circulation. The fluids are absorbed from the raw prostatic surface during resection.

PROSTATITIS

| **What is prostatitis?** | Infection of the prostate gland. May be acute or chronic. |

| **What else can be involved?** | Seminal vesicles and prostatic urethra. |

What are the organisms responsible?	***E. coli*** (main organism) *Staphylococcus aureus* *Streptococcus faecalis* Gonococcus *Chlamydia* (chronic prostatitis).
Where does the infection come from?	Elsewhere via **haematogenous spread** (eg tonsillitis, diverticulitis, etc).
How does the patient present?	**Acute:** high fever, malaise, dysuria, painful defecation, perineal heaviness. **Chronic:** low-grade symptoms of dull ache and referred pain to back and legs; sexual dysfunction; epididymitis; relapsing pyrexia.
What is found on examination?	Exquisitely tender prostate in acute prostatitis (classic finding). In chronic prostatitis, prostate may be tender (not exquisitely) or totally normal.
What are the investigations?	1. MSU for M/C/S 2. Examination of prostatic fluid: fluid gained following prostatic massage (under sedation if necessary) and examined for pus cells 3. Urethroscopy: shows inflammation of prostatic urethra or frank pus from prostatic ducts.
What is the management?	Broad spectrum antibiotics for 10 days pending culture sensitivities (start with a quinolone such as ciprofloxacin), followed by a 4 week course of the appropriate antibiotic (based on sensitivities). **Avoid sex and alcohol for 6 weeks.**
What is the main complication of prostatitis?	Prostatic abscess: must be drained! Use perurethral or perineal route.

d. TESTES, SCROTUM AND PENIS

What are the stages of testicular descent?	**2nd month:** intra-abdominal structure **End of 4th month:** testis at deep inguinal ring. **7th month:** within inguinal canal **Shortly after birth:** within scrotum.
What precedes the testis during descent?	The gubernaculum.
What is the gubernaculum?	A mesenchymal condensation attached to the inferior pole of the testis, whose gradual contraction is thought to drag the testis behind it into the scrotum where it eventually attaches.
What does the testis descend in?	A peritoneal invagination, the **processus vaginalis**.
What is the fate of the processus vaginalis?	Its lumen obliterates shortly after birth, leaving only a small portion surrounding the testis, the **tunica vaginalis**, attached to its posterior and lateral surfaces.
What is the penis made up of?	2 **corpora cavernosa** (sing. corpus cavernosum), the erectile portions of the penis which abut the glans penis. The **glans penis** is the dilated end part of the **corpus spongiosum**, which contains the penile urethra.
What type of epithelium is the penile urethra made up of?	Transitional cell epithelium for most of its length, except for its distal portion which is squamous.

HYDROCELE

What is a hydrocele?	An abnormal collection of fluid in the processus vaginalis.

What types do you know of?	Congenital and acquired.
	Congenital:
	1. **Vaginal:** only the tunica vaginalis part of the processus vaginalis contains fluid (most common)
	2. **Infantile:** fluid fills the processus vaginalis up to the external ring
	3. **Congenital (as well):** the entire processus vaginalis is patent with direct communication between the peritoneal cavity and the scrotum (syn. **congenital hernia**; see below)
	4. **Hydrocele of the cord:** only a discrete portion of the processus vaginalis is patent and fluid-filled.
	Acquired:
	1. Primary or idiopathic
	2. Secondary to testicular disease (eg infection, trauma, carcinoma, TB).
Who gets hydroceles?	Mainly middle-aged and elderly men, despite the hydroceles being of the congenital variety; children and infants get them as well, however.
How does it present?	As a painless scrotal swelling.
How is it differentiated from a hernia clinically?	You can get above it (ie you can palpate the spermatic cord above it); it transilluminates; it has no cough impulse. This differs from a hernia which you *cannot* get above, and which *does* have a cough impulse (unless strangulated).
Which hydrocele is the exception to this rule?	Congenital hydroceles with a fully patent processus vaginalis, hence the alternative name of **congenital herniae.**

How is the diagnosis made?	History, examination and USS. Aspiration of fluid may also be diagnostic, but should not be done before USS is obtained.
What is the treatment?	**Surgical excision:** the hydrocele is incised via a trans-scrotal incision, and drained of its fluid. The empty sac is then invaginated on itself and **marsupialised**, thus preventing re-collection of fluid. This is done via either Lord's or Jabolet's approach.
Why not just aspirate them?	Because of high risk of recurrence (though can be done in the interim while the patient is waiting for an operation, if swelling is big enough to cause discomfort).
What is a haematocele?	A collection of blood in the tunica vaginalis usually due either to trauma or carcinoma. Presents as a bluish scrotal swelling which does not trans-illuminate. Usually self-resolving.
What is a spermatocele?	A cyst arising from the epididymis containing sperm. Aspiration reveals sperm and cinches the diagnosis. Treatment is excision.

VARICOCELE

What is a varicocele?	A collection of dilated (varicosed) veins in the spermatic cord.
Which veins are involved?	The testicular veins, which form the **pampiniform plexus**. This plexus drains the testes to the IVC via the left and right renal vv.
What is thought to cause it?	A defective/absent valve at the junction of the testicular vein and the renal vein, causing backflow of blood and varicosity of the pampiniform plexus.

What side is more commonly affected?	The left side (95%!)
Why?	The angle at which the left testicular v. enters the left renal v. is less acute than on the right.
Who gets it?	Usually presents in teenaged males, but can occur later in life.
How does it present?	It can present as a painless scrotal swelling; there may also be a dragging sensation with dull testicular ache. It may also present as infertility.
What is the classical clinical finding?	Scrotal swelling resembling **a bag of worms**. It may empty on lying flat and does not transilluminate.
Can it cause infertility?	Yes! 40% of infertile men have one.
How does it do this?	Thought to be due to the impaired ability of the veins to deliver heat away from the testis, hence affecting spermatogenesis.
What else can a varicocele cause?	Testicular atrophy (also leading to infertility).
How is it diagnosed?	History, examination and **scrotal USS**.
What is the treatment?	Surgery is the definitive treatment. It involves tying off of the individual varicosed veins of the pampiniform plexus. There are 3 approaches: 1. Open (trans-inguinal) approach (most common) 2. Laparoscopic 3. Percutaneous transvenous: performed by interventional radiologist and reserved for recurrent varicoceles.
Should all varicoceles be operated on?	No.

Why not?	High risk of testicular damage/ atrophy and recurrence.
What are the indications?	1. Symptomatic varicoceles not controlled by analgesia 2. Testicular atrophy 3. Infertility.

FOURNIER'S GANGRENE

What is Fournier's gangrene?	A polymicrobial necrotising fasciitis of the perineal, perianal or genital areas (syn. **idiopathic gangrene of the scrotum**).
Who gets it?	M:F = 10:1
What are the risk factors?	Immunocompromised states (diabetes, steroid use, extremes of age and HIV); urogenital disease (chronic UTI, epididymo-orchitis); alcohol abuse; and cancer. May also be idiopathic.
What are the causative organisms?	*E. coli* (most common aerobe) *Bacterioides* (most common anaerobe) *Proteus* *Staphylococcus aureus* *Enterococcus* *Streptococcus* *Klebsiella* *Clostridium* *Pseudomonas* (There is on average a mixture of 4 organisms.)
How does it present?	Usually as pruritis, followed days after by erythema and swelling with out-of-proportion pain. Necrosis and gangrene eventually (and rapidly) ensue with ↓ pain due to nerve destruction.

What is the precipitating factor?	Usually none, but may follow a minor scratch or bruise to one of the areas above in at-risk patients.
What may occur in Fournier's gangrene if left untreated?	Sloughing of the entire scrotum with full exposure of the testes (which remain disease-free)!
What is the treatment?	1. IV antibiotics: gentamicin and chloramphenicol, pending swab cultures of the affected area 2. Surgical debridement of gangrenous areas, even if testicular exposure is unavoidable (testes can be buried in a tunnel created in the inner thigh on either side, awaiting scrotal reconstruction at a later stage).

PENILE CONDITIONS

What are the indications for circumcision?	1. Religious or cultural reasons (most common) 2. Phimosis/paraphimosis (see below) 3. Recurrent balanitis (infection under prepuce) 4. Torn or tight frenulum.
What is phimosis?	The inability to retract the distal prepuce (foreskin) over the glans penis.
What types of phimosis are there?	Congenital (physiological) and acquired: **Congenital (physiological):** adhesions exist between the prepuce and the glans penis. These adhesions usually resolve by themselves (sometimes by the time the child is a teenager). It does not cause problems such as obstruction.

Acquired: usually due to recurrent balanitis; poor hygiene is a contributing factor.

How can you tell the difference clinically?

In congenital phimosis, the foreskin 'pouts', whereas it does not in acquired phimosis (see Figure 34.2).

What is paraphimosis?

Entrapment of the retracted prepuce behind the coronal sulcus. Causes oedema of the penile head, aggravating the condition. This condition is painful and is a **urological emergency**.

Figure 34.2 Congenital and acquired phimosis

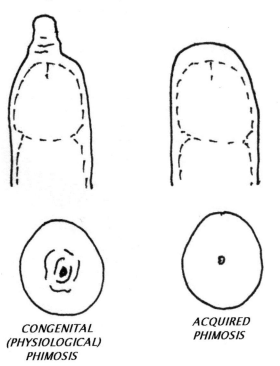

CONGENITAL
(PHYSIOLOGICAL)
PHIMOSIS

ACQUIRED
PHIMOSIS

How is paraphimosis managed?	By firmly squeezing the penile head to empty it of its oedema (anaesthetise the penis first by performing a lignocaine ring block *without* adrenaline), so facilitating reduction of the prepuce. Aspiration of oedema with a large needle (16 G) may be necessary. If all else fails, perform a dorsal slit in the foreskin to release it.
What is priapism?	Persistent, usually painful, erection that lasts for more than four hours. There is no history of sexual stimulation.
What types do you know of?	Low-flow and high-flow. **Low-flow:** results from blood being trapped in the corpus cavernosa (more common). Causes include: 1. Sickle-cell anaemia (common cause; 42% of all adults with sickle-cell will develop it) 2. Drugs: thorazine (anti-depressant) and erectile dysfunction drugs that require intra-cavernous injections 3. Leukaemia 4. Malaria 5. Spinal trauma 6. Carbon monoxide poisoning 7. Marijuana and cocaine 8. Black widow spider bite. **High-flow:** results from arterial rupture causing bleeding within the corpus cavernosa, usually secondary to penile or perineal trauma.
What is seen clinically?	An erect or semi-erect penis with a flaccid glans penis.
What is the treatment?	1. Ice packs may help, followed by aspiration of blood with a large-bore needle.

2. If this fails, intra-cavernous injection of **α-agonists** (eg phenylephrine) which cause arterial constriction, reducing the amount of blood entering penis and allowing time for priapism to subside.
3. A surgical shunt can also be created, shunting blood from the cavernosa.
4. Ligation of ruptured arteries may be necessary in high-flow priapism.

How can the penis be locally anaesthetised for minor surgical procedures?

By use of a ring block with lignocaine *without* adrenaline.

Why without adrenaline?

Adrenaline will cause vasoconstriction of the **end-arteries** which supply the penis, causing penile ischaemia and possible necrosis.

What is Peyronie's disease?

Fibrotic changes in the penis resulting in **plaque formation**, that causes pain, curvature and distortion, usually during erection.

Who gets it?

1% of all men, usually middle-aged.

What is the cause?

Unknown, but *can* develop after penile trauma.

What is the treatment?

Watch and wait: Peyronie's disease may resolve on its own (1–2 years).
Surgery: if not resolving; several options available:
1. Plaque excision and skin graft
2. Plication: 'pinching off' of penile tissue on the opposite side to reduce overall curvature (Nesbit procedure)
3. Penile implant.

CHAPTER 35: SKIN: LUMPS AND BUMPS

How do you describe a skin swelling?

mnemonic: **Should The Children Ever Find Lumps Readily**

Site
Size
Shape
Surface
Symmetry
Skin changes
Temperature
Tenderness
Transilluminability
Transmitted pulsations
Tethering to overlying structures
Consistency (soft, firm, or hard)
Colour
Edge
Expansility
Fluid thrill
Fixed (or mobile)
Lumps elsewhere
Lymph nodes
Resonance.

What are the important points in the history?

1. Painful/painless?
2. Slow/rapidly growing?
3. Duration
4. Sensory/vascular symptoms
5. 'How does this lump affect your life?' Cosmesis, catching on clothes, etc.

What are the principles of management?

Ultimately depends on the type of lump and its site, but based on the following:

1. **Simple excision:** eg for cosmesis as in lipoma
2. **Simple biopsy:** for histological diagnosis in a suspicious lump or bump, where total excision is not immediately possible (eg ulcer edge)

3. **Excision biopsy:** for histological diagnosis in a suspicious lump or bump which can *also* be fully excised at the same time (eg lymph node)
4. **Wide local excision:** if simple biopsy reveals malignancy, total clearance of the lump with safe margins is undertaken (eg skin cancers)
5. **Lymph node clearance:** done if disease has spread to the lymph drainage of a malignant lump (eg melanoma)
6. **Radiotherapy:** appropriate to the affected lump or its lymph drainage area if the tumour is radiosensitive (eg melanoma or breast cancer).

How would you describe an ulcer?

1. Size
2. Shape
3. Position
4. Edge:
    *   Flat (venous)
    *   Punched-out and squared (syphilis or diabetic [trophic])
    *   Sloping (healing)
    *   Undermined (pressure, TB)
    *   Rolled (basal cell carcinoma)
    *   Everted (squamous cell carcinoma).
5. Base (eg dry, sloughy)
6. Discharge
7. Surrounding tissue
8. Local nerve and blood supply
9. Regional lymph nodes.

What are the most common lumps and bumps?

See Table 35.1.

Table 35.1

Lesion (Benign unless stated)	Layer from which lesion is derived	Most common site for lesion	Size	Appearance (diameter)	Treatment
Skin tag	Epidermis	Trunk, neck, axillae, groin	Up to 5 mm	Loose connective tissue covered by normal, often pigmented keratinised epithelium	Cautery/ excision
Warts	Epidermis	Fingers and back of hands	Up to 1 cm	Depends on location	Keratolytic application/ cryosurgery
Seborrhoeic keratosis	Epidermis	Chest, face, neck, arms	Up to several cm	Slightly raised, sharply demarcated, plaque-like	'Scraped off' with a curette
Keratoacanthoma	Epidermis	Varies	Up to 2 cm	Nodular with a central keratin plug	Local excision
Solar keratosis (premalignant)	Epidermis	Sun-exposed areas	Variable	Flat, well-demarcated, brown, crusty, with erythematous base	Depends on history, excised usually
Squamous cell carcinoma (malignant)	Epidermis	Anywhere on the skin	Variable	Enlarging ulcer with rolled indurated margin, or cauliflower-like appearance	Biopsy – radiotherapy/ excision + margin
Basal cell carcinoma (malignant)	Epidermis	Usually upper part of the face	Variable	Start as pearly-white nodules with visible vessels. May ulcerate	Radiotherapy, cryotherapy, or curettage
Intradermal naevus	Melanocytes of epidermal layer	Everywhere except palm, sole of foot, or scrotum	Variable	Light/dark, flat/raised, hairy/hairless	None

Table 35.1 (continued)

Junctional naevus	Melanocytes of epidermal layer	Anywhere	Variable	Flat, smooth and hairless	None – unless leads to malignancy
Compound naevus	Melanocytes of epidermal layer	Anywhere	Variable	Slightly raised/ moderately pigmented	None – unless leads to malignancy
Malignant melanoma	Melanocytes of epidermal layer	Sun-exposed areas	Variable	Black/ dark-brown, flat/nodular, bleed/ulcerate	See Chapter 49
Pyogenic granuloma	Dermis	Hands and feet	Develops over approx. one week	Solitary, reddish-blue fleshy nodules	Excised with the base curetted or cauterised
Histiocytoma/ dermatofibroma	Dermis	Limbs	Approx. 5 mm	Reddish-brown. May look similar to malignant melanoma	None
Kaposi's sarcoma (malignant)	Dermis	Limbs	Variable	Blueish-red to brown nodules or plaques	Excision biopsy
Furuncle (boil)	Dermis	Back of trunk and lower limbs	Variable	Abscess in hair follicle	Usually spontaneously heals
Carbuncle	Dermis	Back of neck	Larger than furuncles	Multilocular abscess draining via multiple sinuses	Antibiotics plus drainage
Epidermal cysts (sebaceous cysts)	Epidermis	Scalp, trunk, face and neck	Up to several cm	Smooth and rounded and covered by normal epidermis. Punctum may be visible. May contain sebum	Excision if history of infection present
Dermoid cysts	Dermis	Midline of scalp, neck and lower jaw	Up to several cm	Cystic swelling	Excision

Table 35.1 (continued)

Pilonidal sinus	Dermis	Skin of natal cleft	Variable	Solitary sinus or may appear as a row in the midline	If abscess present – drainage
Lipoma	Hypodermis	Forearms and supra-clavicular fossa	2–20 cm	Soft, lobulated and fluctuant	Excision for cosmesis
Neurofibroma	Peripheral nerves	Anywhere on the integument	Variable	Soft, pedunculated, mobile from side to side	Enucleation or resection
Ganglion (pl. ganglia)	Lining of synovial joint, tendon sheath, or embryological remnants	Wrist, dorsum of foot, or along flexor aspect of fingers and on the peroneal tendons	1–2 cm	Cystic, sub-cutaneous, pea-sized lump	Excision for cosmesis
Cystic hygroma	Jugular lymph sac in neck	Neck	Can grow extremely large	Soft, fluctuant, highly trans-illuminable	Difficult to excise

What is the 'slip sign'?

In examining a lipoma, the edge can be felt to 'slip' under your fingers: characteristic of a lipoma!

Does a lipoma have malignant potential?

No! Liposarcoma is a separate entity.

What is Dercum's disease?

Multiple, painful lipomatosis (mainly truncal).

What is characteristic of lumps from tubular/cord-like structures such as vessels or nerves?

They move in **1 plane only,** ie the plane **arising** perpendicular to the structure to which they are attached. Other lumps move in more than one plane.

Do ganglia communicate with the joint space?

No. They arise from the **joint lining** and are completely separate. A lump which communicates with the joint space is capsular herniation.

What was the old-fashioned way of treating a ganglion?

Whacking it with the family Bible!

What is an ulcer?

A break in the continuity of an epithelial surface.

What is Cock's peculiar tumour?

An ulcerated sebaceous cyst of the scalp.
Rx: excision biopsy to r/o malignancy.

What is an ivory osteoma?

A slowly-growing, ivory-hard benign tumour arising from the cortical layer of the flat bones of the skull, face and orbit. (Exam oddity!)
Rx: simple excision.

What is characteristic of a sebaceous cyst?

The presence of a **punctum**, a tiny hole through which sebum drains (not always present!).

What is a ranula?

A transparent **retention cyst** in the floor of the mouth arising from the sublingual salivary glands. Ranula means a small frog in Latin, and the cyst is so-called because of a supposed resemblance to a small frog!

How are neck lumps classified?

Into 2 categories:
1. Midline and non-midline lumps.
2. Anterior or posterior neck triangle.

What are the boundaries of the neck triangles?

Anterior: midline (imaginary line), mandible and the anterior border of sternocleidomastoid (SCM).
Posterior: posterior border of SCM, anterior border of trapezius and the clavicle.

Which nerve is in danger of being damaged during excision of a lump in the posterior triangle?

Spinal accessory nerve (CN XI).

What are its landmarks?

It runs from the posterior border of the junction of the upper and middle thirds of SCM to the anterior border of the junction of the middle and lower thirds of trapezius.

What does its damage result in?

Difficulty in shrugging ipsilateral shoulder (trapezius weakness) and turning head to opposite side (SCM weakness).

What is the differential diagnosis of a midline neck lump?

1. Thyroid mass
2. Thyroglossal cyst
3. Lipoma
4. Sebaceous cyst.

What is a branchial cyst?

A lump which arises from embryonic remnants of the second branchial cleft in the neck. It is most common in young adults where it presents as a smooth swelling in front of the anterior border of the SCM at the **junction of its upper and middle thirds.** The position is characteristic.

C. Surgical malignancy

CHAPER 36: OESOPHAGEAL CARCINOMA

What is the incidence of oesophageal cancer?

15:100,000
Male:Female ratio 3:1.

What is the most common type of oesophageal cancer?

The majority of oesophageal malignancies are **squamous cell carcinomas**. However, the distal 2 cm of the oesophagus is lined with **columnar epithelium** and a small number of **adenocarcinomas** can arise here.

What is Barrett's oesophagus?

Metaplasia of the naturally occurring squamous cell epithelium into columnar epithelium caused by the chronic irritation of the epithelium by acid reflux.

What is its significance?

80% (40-fold) increased risk of **adenocarcinoma** developing subsequently. Patients require close endoscopic monitoring (see Chapter 29a).

What are the risk factors associated with oesophageal cancer?

1. GORD (causing **Barrett's oesophagus**)
2. Achalasia
3. Diet (especially pickled/preserved food)
4. Corrosives (eg lye ingestion)
5. Smoking
6. Alcohol
7. Plummer–Vinson syndrome (post-cricoid oesophageal web 2ry to iron deficiency anaemia, presenting as dysphagia; web is prone to carcinomatous change)
8. Familial link ($\uparrow$ in Chinese).

How can risk factors also be remembered?

mnemonic: **ABCDEF**
Achalasia
Barrett's oesophagus
Corrosives

Diet
oEsophageal webs
Familial.

How does it present?

Dysphagia (classically **painless and progressive**)
Odynophagia
Weight loss
Regurgitation
Symptoms of anaemia (eg pallor, fatigue)
Symptoms of metastatic disease (eg jaundice, ascites, lymphadenopathy, chest pain)
Cough
Recurrent chest infections.

What are the investigations?

Blood investigations:
FBC: anaemia
LFTs: deranged if liver mets present
Clotting: also deranged in liver involvement
Imaging:
CXR: may show aspiration pneumonia, lung mets, pleural effusions, hilar lymphadenopathy
Ba swallow: gives anatomical detail of cancer (classically **rat-tail appearance**)
CT scan: used for staging the disease ie mets and lymphadenopathy.
Trans-oesophageal ultrasound (TOE): useful for assessing the degree of local invasion of the tumour
Endoscopy:
Gold standard; lesions can be directly visualised and biopsied for a tissue diagnosis.

How is it managed?

Only 30% of oesophageal tumours are operable as many patients

present at a late stage. Treatment is therefore aimed mainly towards **palliation** and **symptom relief**.

Surgery: only appropriate for a small number of patients where the tumour is resectable. The oesophagus is either rejoined or connected distally to the stomach.

Chemo/radiotherapy: has a limited role in but has been increasingly used as a means of neoadjuvant therapy (given prior to surgery).

Endoscopy: strictures can be dilated endoscopically with/without placements of stents to relieve dysphagia. **Laser ablation** of the tumour can also be performed endoscopically.

Analgesia and **nutritional support** form a large part in palliative care.

What is the prognosis?

Overall prognosis is poor. 5-year survival rates 5%, and only 15% with resection.

CHAPTER 37: GASTRIC CARCINOMA

What is the incidence of gastric cancer?

M:F ratio 2:1
High incidence in Japan, Chile and Eastern Europe

What types of gastric cancer are there?

The majority are **adenocarcinomas** (>90%) arising from the normal glandular epithelium of the stomach. Other malignant tumours may occur but are relatively rare eg neuroendocrine 5-HT secreting tumours and lymphomas.

What is the most common site for GI lymphomas to occur?

The stomach.

Where do carcinomas arise within the stomach?

60% antrum, 25% fundus, 15% body.

What is the Lauren Classification?

A histological classification of gastric cancers
Cancers are either **intestinal-type** or **diffuse**.
Intestinal-type: resembles glandular tissue and invades as an expanding mass.
Diffuse: made up of single or small groups of cells. **Has a worse prognosis.**

How do gastric cancers spread?

Locally: if the tumour extends beyond the **serosa** there is a risk of peritoneal dissemination and invasion into adjacent organs eg pancreas, liver or spleen.
Lymphatic: local node involvement initially, and then more distantly eg supraclavicular nodes (Syn.: **Virchow's nodes**).
Haematogenous: spread via the portal vein causing liver metastases (common in advanced disease).

Transcoelomic: this means spread through peritoneal cavity; occurs most commonly to the ovaries (Syn.: **Krukenberg tumours**).

What are the risk factors?

1. Pernicious anaemia
2. *H. pylori* infection (especially in lymphomas)
3. Gastric ulcers
4. History of gastric surgery
5. Adenomatous polyps
6. Diet, especially spicy or salty foods
7. Alcohol
8. Smoking
9. Blood group A
10. Positive family history.

What symptoms do patients commonly present with?

Weight loss
Dyspepsia
Anorexia
Post-prandial fullness (2ry to mass effect of tumour)
Dysphagia (esp. with oesophageal extension)
Vomiting
Symptoms of iron deficiency anaemia (eg fatigue, pallor)
Symptoms of metastatic disease (eg jaundice, back pain).

What would you find on examination?

Oftentimes nothing during the early stages of disease. Late presenters may have the following:
General: cachexia
Hands: pallor and koilonychias of nails (anaemia)
Face: pale mucous membranes, jaundice
Neck: lymphadenopathy, in particular **Virchow's node** in the left supraclavicular fossa (**Troisier's sign**).

Chest: pleural effusions (2ry to chest mets)
Abdomen: epigastric mass, hepatomegaly (liver mets), ascites (peritoneal mets), **Sister Mary Joseph sign** (umbilical mets)
Rectum: rectal shelf (mass felt anteriorly on rectal exam 2ry to peritoneal mets in the pouch of Douglas; syn. **Bloomer's shelf**).

What are the investigations?	**Blood investigations:**

1. FBC: anaemia
2. U&Es: baseline assessment; may be deranged in malnutrition
3. LFTs: assessment of jaundice if present; may be deranged in liver involvement
4. Clotting: may be deranged in liver involvement
5. Bone profile: may be deranged in bone mets.

Imaging:
1. CXR: for staging of cancer (chest mets) and assessing patient's operative state
2. Abdominal USS: staging (tumour assessment)
3. CT chest and abdomen: staging (mets and lymph node spread).

Endoscopy: gold standard; may reveal areas of bleeding, ulcerated surfaces, or mass lesions. Any area of abnormality should be biopsied allowing a histological diagnosis to be made.

What is the management?

Usually **palliative** as patients often present in the late stages of disease with inoperable tumours. If surgery *is* considered, pt. must be medically optimised.

When is the role of surgery?

If the patient is optimised medically, then surgery is more likely to be curative if disease is localised ie confined to the serosa, and has a clearly demarcated margin. Surgery may also play a palliative role (see below).

What is the role of surgery in gastric cancer?

Curative or palliative.

Curative: tumour is confined to the serosa and has a clearly demarcated margin. A **total gastrectomy** is performed, with anastomosis of the distal end of the oesophagus to a loop of small bowel for continuity (**Roux-en-Y** procedure; see Figure 29.4, p. 238). A **partial gastrectomy** can also be performed.

Palliative: tumour is inoperable. Surgery is performed to achieve symptom control for the patient rather than improving mortality. Symptoms that can be alleviated include nausea, vomiting and dysphagia. Nutrition may also be improved by bypassing an obstructing tumour

Procedures include:

1. Palliative resection of an obstructing tumour
2. Bypass of tumour (gastroenterostomy)
3. Stents or endoscopic laser therapy (bypass or down-size tumour respectively).

What other measures are there?

Blood transfusions for symptomatic anaemia. Limited role for chemo/radiotherapy but may induce regression in susceptible patients.

What is the most important prognostic factor?

The number of affected lymph nodes (hence importance of staging these patients). 5-year survival rates fall from 95% (if the tumour is respectable and no nodal involvement) to 5% (nodal involvement present).

CHAPTER 38: SMALL BOWEL CARCINOMA

How common is small bowel carcinoma?

Not common at all. It is *rare*.

What percentage of bowel malignancies does it represent?

Less than 1%.

Which part of the small bowel is most commonly affected?

Duodenum > jejunum > ileum.

What are the risk factors?

1. Coeliac disease (risk of lymphoma)
2. Hereditary bowel syndromes (FAP, HNPCC, Peutz–Jegher syndrome).

What is Peutz–Jegher syndrome?

Syndrome of benign GI polyps with circumoral pigmentation.

What is the most common 1ry small bowel cancer?

Adenocarcinoma (40%).

How does small bowel cancer present?

Late due to non-specific symptoms and low index of suspicion due to its rarity. May occasionally present as anaemia, obstruction or intussusception.

What are the investigations?

Barium follow-through (shows luminal filling defect) and CT scan. However, both have poor sensitivity for small bowel cancer. CT is important in staging of the disease.

What is the treatment?

Resection of the tumour. Adjuvant therapy is as for colorectal carcinoma (see p. 371) in adenocarcinoma.

CHAPTER 39: LARGE BOWEL CARCINOMA: COLORECTAL AND ANAL

What is colorectal carcinoma?

Adenocarcinoma affecting the colon and/or rectum.

Which part of the large bowel is most commonly affected?

The rectum (50%).

What is its incidence?

2nd most common cancer in UK with a M:F ratio of 1:1. Risk begins in the 40s and peaks in the 7th decade of life.

What are the risk factors?

1. Diet rich in fat and cholesterol
2. Ulcerative colitis
3. Adenomatous polyps (esp. **villous adenoma**; see Chapter 30a)
4. Familial predisposition:
   a. Family history of colorectal cancer (known as hereditary non-polyposis colon cancer [HNPCC])
   b. Familial adenomatous polyposis syndromes (see Chapter 30a)
5. Previous colorectal cancer (**metachronous risk**)
6. Pre-existing cancer (**synchronous risk**).

What are the complications of colorectal cancer?

1. Stricture formation and resultant large bowel obstruction (see Chapter 18)
2. Perforation (most common in caecum) and resultant faecal peritonitis (see Chapter 18)
3. Fistula formation (see Chapter 3)
4. Lower GI bleed (see Chapter 21).

How are large bowel tumours broadly classified?

As **right-sided** (caecum, ascending and proximal transverse colon) and **left-sided** (distal transverse, descending and sigmoid colon and rectum) tumours.

How do they present?

Right-sided tumours: weight loss, and symptoms of anaemia (fatigue, headache, palpitations) 2ry to occult blood in the stool.
Left-sided tumours: abdominal pain, altered bowel habit and rectal bleeding (classically mixed in with stool, but may be bright red if low-lying). May present initially as a large bowel obstruction (see Chapter 18), or a perforation with peritonitis.

What are the clinical findings?

General: signs of Fe-deficiency anaemia (pale mucous membranes, koilonychia); cachexia; jaundice if liver involvement; left supraclavicular (Virchow's) nodes.
Abdominal: look for scars from previous surgery (?prior cancer); a LIF or RIF mass may be palpable; hepatomegaly if liver mets; ascites if peritoneal seeding.
Rectal: low-lying tumour may be palpable; feel for rectal shelf secondary to peritoneal seeding and carcinomatous deposits in the pouch of Douglas (Bloomer's sign); there may be blood on the glove (commonly altered, but may be bright red if tumour is low-lying).
Systems: chest examination for pleural effusion in lung mets.

How does it spread?

Lymphatic: to regional lymph nodes (mesenteric), then on to para-aortic nodes and the thoracic duct.
Haematogenous: mainly to the liver (via portal vein), but also to the lungs, adrenal glands, kidneys and bones.

Trans-coelomic: also known as peritoneal seeding, it can spread to the ovaries (**Krukenburg tumour**).

What are the investigations?

Blood investigations:
1. FBC: anaemia
2. U&Es: baseline; electrolyte imbalance in cachexia
3. LFTs: raised in liver mets; albumin low if malnourished
4. Clotting screen: may be abnormal in liver involvement
5. Tumour marker: carcinoembryonic antigen (CEA); important in response to treatment or detecting recurrence so take pre-operative sample.

Imaging:
1. **CXR:** r/o pleural effusion and lung mets
2. **Endoscopy:** the following in sequence should be performed:
   i.   Rigid sigmoidoscopy
   ii. Flexible sigmoidoscopy
   iii. Colonoscopy.
3. **Contrast study:** double-contrast Ba enema (do single-contrast if pt. presents as obstruction).
4. **CT scan:** chest, abdomen and pelvis for staging.

What else can cause a raised CEA?

Hepatobiliary and pancreatic disease, so correlate raised CEA results with CT scan and colonoscopic findings.

How is colorectal cancer staged?

With the **Dukes classification:**
Stage A: carcinoma *in situ* limited to mucosa or submucosa
Stage B1: cancer extends into the muscularis
Stage B2: cancer extends into or through the serosa
Stage C: cancer extends to regional lymph nodes

Stage D: cancer has metastasised to distant sites (modified classification; stage D was not in the original Dukes classification).

Figure 39.1 Dukes classification of colorectal disease

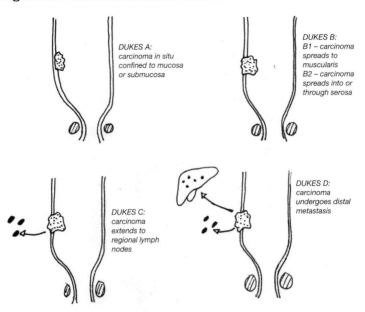

DUKES A:
carcinoma in situ
confined to mucosa
or submucosa

DUKES B:
B1 – carcinoma
spreads to
muscularis
B2 – carcinoma
spreads into or
through serosa

DUKES C:
carcinoma
extends to
regional lymph
nodes

DUKES D:
carcinoma
undergoes distal
metastasis

What is the management?

Based on treatment of the tumour (surgery) and treatment of its spread (adjuvant therapy). Management is therefore based on the Dukes stage.

How is the tumour managed?

This depends on the area of large bowel involved:
Right hemicolectomy: caecum or ascending colon up to hepatic flexure.
Extended right hemicolectomy: transverse colon.
Left hemicolectomy: descending colon distal to splenic flexure.

High anterior resection: sigmoid colon.
Anterior resection: upper rectum
Abdomino-perineal resection (APR): lower rectum.
Panproctocolectomy: FAP coli or UC.

Is a stoma fashioned routinely?	No. Primary anastomosis of the bowel ends is usually possible following excision of the tumour.

When would you consider stoma formation?

1. If primary anastomosis is <12 cm from anal verge (eg low rectal tumours): high risk of anastomotic breakdown (perform a **defunctioning ileostomy** to allow bowel to rest and anastomosis to heal).
2. If presentation is not an elective one (eg pt. presents as large bowel obstruction or perforation of tumour): also high risk of anastomotic breakdown (perform a **defunctioning colostomy**).

Anastomosis of the ends can be carried out in both of these as a second procedure at 6 weeks with reversal of the stoma.

3. If an APR is being performed (perform a **permanent colostomy**; see below).

What is an anterior resection?

Removal of the part of the diseased sigmoid colon or rectum via a low abdominal (anterior) incision.

What is an APR?

Removal of a low rectal tumour involving mobilisation of the rectum via a combined abdominal (anterior) and perineal approach. The anal opening is usually sutured closed in the process, necessitating the need for a permanent stoma.

What must be done prior to surgery?	Bowel prep.
What does this entail?	In **elective** cases: 3 days liquid-only diet and a laxative 24 hours before surgery. In **emergency** cases: on-table colonic lavage. *All* cases should receive antibiotics at induction and post-op (see your hospital policy).
What is the rule of thumb during tumour resection in the bowel?	Resect the tumour with 5 cm disease free margins proximally and distally.
What are the adjuvant modalities?	May be either radio- or chemotherapy. **Radiotherapy:** used in rectal cancer; avoided in colon cancer due to high incidence of post-irradiation adhesions. Its main goal in rectal cancer is the **prevention of recurrence**. It is given either pre- or post-op. Success ↑ if given in combo with chemotherapy. **Chemotherapy:** used in both colonic and rectal cancer. Effect on survival: Dukes A: not indicated as no improvement Dukes B: unclear Dukes C/D: definite improvement **5-fluorouracil (5FU)** is used.
What must be given with 5FU?	Folinic acid, which prevents myelosuppression caused by 5FU (**folinic acid rescue**).
What is the prognosis?	Dukes A 5-year survival rate is 90% following resection; Dukes B is 75–80% following resection with or without adjuvant therapy; Dukes C is 30–60% following resection and adjuvant therapy; Dukes D is poor at 5%.

Who should be screened for colorectal cancer?	1. Long-standing UC 2. Familial adenomatous polyposis syndromes 3. HNPCC 4. Previous colorectal cancer (metachronous cancers) 5. History of adenomatous polyps.
How is screening carried out?	Two methods in use: 1. **Faecal occult blood test (FOBT):** stool smeared on a card and impregnated with guaiac acid; H_2O_2 is added to it in the lab and a colour change indicates blood present. False positives are seen in patients on Fe supplements and those who have recently eaten red meat. 2. **Flexible sigmoidoscopy:** direct vision possible, as is biopsy, but entire colon cannot be tested. Not acceptable to all patients as it is invasive.

ANAL CARCINOMA

What is the most common type of anal cancer?	Squamous cell carcinoma (80%).
What others can occur?	1. Adenocarcinoma (from anal glands) 2. Malignant melanoma (see Chapter 49) 3. Kaposi's sarcoma.
What are the risk factors?	1. Anal sex 2. Genital warts (HPV).
What is the aetiology?	Homosexuals are more prone; usually presents in 40–50 year olds.
How does it present?	As a painful, bleeding anal lump.

What are the differentials?	It must be distinguished from the following: 1. Haemorrhoids 2. Perianal haematoma 3. Anal fissure 4. Anal warts.
What are the clinical findings?	An anal mass which is usually fungating (exophytic), though may present as an ulcerating lesion. There may be bleeding. Inguinal lymph nodes may be palpable in spread.
What *must* be done on examination?	Proctoscopy to rule out anal *canal* lesions as opposed to anal verge lesions only.
What are the investigations?	Examination under anaesthesia should be done with biopsy of the lesion.
What is the management?	**Local excision:** if lesion is <2 cm diameter **Radiotherapy:** usual mode of treatment; external beam radiotherapy is applied to lesion and affected nodes if involved. **APR:** reserved for aggressive tumours; permanent colostomy is necessary.

CHAPTER 40: PANCREATIC CARCINOMA

What is pancreatic carcinoma?
A common, fatal, metastasising adenocarcinoma of the pancreatic ducts.

What is its incidence?
4th most common cancer in UK, affecting males more than females (3:2), with a peak incidence at ages 60–80.

What are the risk factors?
1. Smoking
2. Diabetes
3. Caffeine
4. Heavy alcohol use
5. FAP
6. Gardner's syndrome.

What parts of the pancreas are affected?
Head (70%), body (20%), tail (10%).

How does it present?
History can be vague, but generally depends on the part affected:
Head: **Painless jaundice** (classic sign; due to bile duct obstruction), pruritis, distended gallbladder (as per **Courvoisier's law**) and weight loss.
Body and tail: Weight loss and **pain** with migratory thrombophlebitis (**Trousseau's sign**).
Jaundice occurs in <10% of cases.

What in the history makes one suspicious of a diagnosis of pancreatic carcinoma?
1. Upper abdominal backache with negative USS and endoscopy
2. Unexplained weight loss
3. Pancreatitis in absence of gallstones
4. Newly diagnosed diabetic with dyspepsia.

Investigations?
Blood investigations:
1. FBC: ↓Hb
2. LFT: investigation of obstructive jaundice

3. Clotting: may be deranged in long standing obstructive jaundice.

Radiology:
1. USS: visualise tumour and r/o gallstones in jaundiced patient
2. CT scan: good tumour imaging and useful in staging
3. ERCP: possible biopsy/brushings
4. Selective angiography: for staging and defining a. and v. involvement and anatomy.

What is the treatment?

Surgical: depends on location of tumour.
Head: **Whipple's procedure** (see below)
Body/tail: distal pancreatic resection.
Palliative: in incurable disease to alleviate problems such as:
- Obstructive jaundice (common bile duct stenting)
- Pain (chemical splanchnectomy)
- Duodenal obstruction (bypass procedures such as gastrojejunostomy).

What is Whipple's procedure?

A pancreaticoduodenectomy. The following steps are involved (in order):
1. Cholecystectomy (removal of gallbladder)
2. Truncal vagotomy (denervation of stomach)
3. Antrectomy (resection of stomach antrum)
4. Pancreaticoduodenectomy (removal of head of pancreas and duodenum)
5. Choledochojejunostomy (anastomosis of biliary duct to jejunum)
6. Pancreaticojejunostomy (anastomosis of pancreatic remnant to jejunum)

7. Gastrojejunostomy (anastomosis of stomach remnant to jejunum).
    End result is shown in Figure 40.1.

Figure 40.1 End result after Whipple's procedure

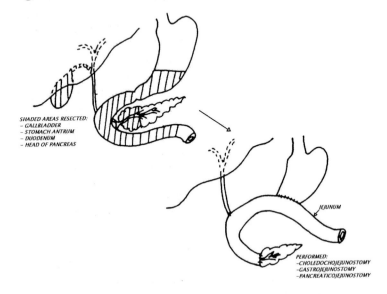

SHADED AREAS RESECTED:
– GALLBLADDER
– STOMACH ANTRUM
– DUODENUM
– HEAD OF PANCREAS

JEJUNUM

PERFORMED:
–CHOLEDOCHOJEJUNOSTOMY
–GASTROJEJUNOSTOMY
–PANCREATICOJEJUNOSTOMY

What is the prognosis?

Poor. 90% die within 1 year of diagnosis.
Average survival rate is 5–15% @ 5 years post-resection.

CHAPTER 41: HEPATIC CARCINOMA

What types of liver cancers do you know?

Primary and secondary.

Which type is more common?

Secondary (ie metastasis of another primary cancer to the liver, known as **metastatic liver disease**). 20 times more common than 1ry cancer!

What are the types of primary liver cancer?

They include:
1. **Hepatocellular carcinoma**: most common of the 1ry cancers (but still less common than 2ry cancer); arises from hepatocytes (syn. **hepatoma**, a misnomer).
2. **Cholangiocarcinoma**: arises from small bile ducts in the liver.
3. **Angiosarcoma**: asrise from hepatic vessels
4. **Hepatoblastoma**: rare tumour occurring in children.

Which one is the most common?

Hepatocellular carcinoma (75%); 2ry cancer still more common overall!

What are the risk factors of 1ry liver cancer?

1. Hepatitis B & C
2. Cirrhosis
3. Vinyl chloride in the plastic industry, arsenic, Thorotrast contrast (all cause angiosarcoma)
4. Hepatocellular adenoma
5. Ulcerative colitis
6. Primary biliary cirrhosis (increase the risk of cholangiocarcinoma)
7. Glycogen storage disease type 1
8. Aflatoxins: occur in food contaminated with *Aspergillus flavus* (eg mouldy nuts).

How does the patient present?

Late presentation: weight loss, loss of appetite, nausea and vomiting, abdominal pain in the right hypochondrium radiating to the back (stretching of Glisson's capsule).

What are the relevant points in the history?

1. Tattoos, IVDU, sexual history, travel history and transfusions (hepatitis B & C)
2. Alcohol history (cirrhosis)
3. Occupational history (plastic industry)
4. Past medical history:
   a. Cirrhosis (Wilson's disease, α1-antitrypsin deficiency, haemochromatosis)
   b. 1ry biliary cirrhosis
   c. Ulcerative colitis
   d. Glycogen storage disease
   e. Other cancers (possibility of metastatic disease).
5. Drug history: OCP, anabolic steroids (↑risk of hepatocellular adenoma)
6. Exposure to aflatoxin.

What are the signs?

Signs are not specific for liver cancer but more of general liver disease. They tend to appear late:
General: cachexia, jaundice.
Hands: specific to disease process (eg cirrhosis, IBD if present).
Abdomen: palpable liver (liver mets are classically hard and craggy, giving the liver an irregular edge; liver may be impalpable if cirrhosis is the cause); ascites.

NB As 2ry liver cancer is most common, there will usually be signs of the 1ry disease (eg colorectal cancer, breast cancer, IBD). *A full head to toe examination of all systems is therefore warranted!* See relevant chapters for specific signs.

What are the investigations?	**Blood investigations:**
	FBC: anaemia of chronic disorder
	LFTs: ↑ALP, ↑ALT, ↑AST, ↑γGT, ↑bilirubin (hence jaundice), ↓albumin
	Clotting screen: may be ↓ 2ry to ↓clotting factor production
	Tumour markers: for 1ry tumour if suspected (eg CEA for colon cancer). α-fetoprotein (AFP) may be raised in 1ry liver cancer, but is non-specific.
	Imaging:
	USS: can be used to visualise the liver and take guided biopsies.
	CT scan: plain and contrast will show size and pattern of tumour. CT-guided biopsies can also be taken.
	MRI: bile ducts can be visualised; important esp. in cholangiocarcinoma.
	Angiography: of the coeliac axis or superior mesenteric vessels can be used to assess the vascularity of the tumour.
What is the treatment?	**Surgical:** up to 80% of the liver can be resected. Post-resection, the 5-year survival rate is 25%. If there is no extrahepatic spread, then a transplant can be considered.
	Adjunctive: both chemo- and radiotherapy have been shown to have disappointing results.
	Palliative: symptomatic relief if tumour unresectable. Survival rate in these patients is <1 year.

CHAPTER 42: GALLBLADDER AND BILIARY TREE CARCINOMA

GALLBLADDER CARCINOMA

What type of cancer is it?	An adenocarcinoma.
What is its claim to fame?	Most common 1ry hepatobiliary cancer (still rare though!)
Who gets it?	F:M = 3:1, more common in ages > 65.
What are its risk factors?	1. Long-standing cholelithiasis (esp. cholesterol stones) 2. Porcelain gallbladder (see Chapter 29e) 3. Family history 4. Infection by *Salmonella typhi* 5. Anomalous pancreaticobiliary duct junction (irritation from pancreatic juice reflux).
How does it present?	Usually asymptomatic. Gallbladder is removed for other reasons (eg cholelithiasis), and carcinoma found incidentally on histology. For this reason it usually presents **late**. Spread may result in: 1. Obstructive jaundice (local spread to biliary tree) 2. Hepatomegaly (spread to liver) 3. Cholecystoenteric fistula.
What are the investigations?	**Blood investigations:** raised LFTs (mainly ALP) **Imaging:** 1. **AXR:** gallstones, porcelain gallbladder, air cholecystogram (2ry to cholecystoenteric fistula) 2. **USS:** most commonly used; shows gallbladder wall thickening, intraluminal masses, and irregular echogenicity

3. **CT scan:** shows tumour (**jam-packed gallbladder:** entire lumen full of tumour), plus important for staging (extent of spread, lymph node involvement, mets).

How is it managed?

Surgical excision. With early disease (confined to gallbladder wall), cholecystectomy is curative (90–96%). With spread, tumour excision with clear margins is performed.

What is the prognosis?

Overall poor.

CHOLANGIOCARCINOMA

What is cholangiocarcinoma?

Carcinoma of the biliary tree.

What parts of the tree are affected?

Anywhere from the originating biliary ducts in the liver to the ampulla of Vater.

What type of cancer is it?

Adenocarcinoma (95%), squamous cell carcinoma (5%).

Who gets them?

M:F = 1.5:1; pts aged 60 most likely to have it; Japanese have the highest incidence worldwide.

What are the causes?

1. IBD (UC>Crohn's)
2. Congenital cysts of the biliary tree (choledochal cysts and Caroli disease)
3. Sclerosing cholangitis
4. Infection with liver flukes (*Clonorchis sinensis* and *Opisthorcis viverrini*)
5. Chemical exposure (aircraft, wood-finishing and rubber industries; Thorotrast contrast medium; ?agent orange).

How do they present?	Weight loss and symptoms of obstructive jaundice (see Chapter 29e).

What are the investigations?	**Blood investigations:** raised LFTs (mainly ALP); investigate as for obstructive jaundice if present.
	Imaging:
	1. **USS:** study of choice; shows larger tumours and biliary dilation.
	2. **CT:** shows tumour; important in staging.
	3. **ERCP:** has the following advantages:
	  a. Clearly delineates biliary tree; tumour appears as a filling defect
	  b. Biliary tree brushings can be sent for cytology
	  c. Palliative stenting may relieve obstructive jaundice.

What is a Klatskin tumour?	Cholangiocarcinoma involving the junction of the right and left hepatic ducts.
What is the management of cholangiocarcinoma?	Depends on the level of occurrence in the biliary tree: **Proximal:** tumour resection with hepaticojejunostomy (anastomosis of hepatic bile ducts to the jejunum) **Distal:** Whipple's procedure (see Chapter 40).
What is the prognosis?	Generally poor.
What risks can complicate cholangiocarcinoma?	Obstructive jaundice and ascending cholangitis.
What is Caroli disease?	Caroli disease/syndrome is a rare congenital disorder of the intrahepatic bile ducts. It is characterised by intrahepatic dilatation of the biliary tree.

What is it associated with?

Autosomal dominant polycystic kidney disease.

Who is Caroli disease more common in?

Females.

CHAPTER 43: BREAST CANCER

APPLIED ANATOMY

What is the lymphatic drainage of the breast?

75% drainage to the axilla; 25% to the internal mammary nodes (2nd–4th intercostal spaces).

What are the boundaries of the axilla?

Anterior wall: pectoralis major and minor, subclavius and clavipectoral fascia.
Posterior wall: subscapularis and teres major
Medial wall: upper part of serratus anterior down to the level of the 4th rib.
Lateral wall: anterior and posterior walls converging at humeral bicipital groove
Apex: bounded by clavicle, scapula, and 1st rib
Floor: axillary fascia, subcutaneous tissue and skin.

What are the contents of the axilla?

1. Axillary artery
2. Axillary vein
3. Brachial plexus
4. Lymph nodes.

What groups of nodes are in the axilla?

Anatomically, 5 groups in all: anterior, posterior, lateral, central and apical. The axillary nodes can also be grouped **clinically** into level I, II and III nodes depending on whether they are lateral, posterior, or medial to **pectoralis minor** respectively.

CLINICAL CONSIDERATIONS

What is the incidence of breast cancer?

26 per 100,000 females in the UK. Breast cancer is the number one malignancy affecting women in the Western world.

Can men be affected?	**Yes!** However, much less common, accounting for 1% of all breast cancer cases and is associated with a worse prognosis (less breast tissue, hence faster invasion by time of presentation).
What is the difference between carcinoma-in-situ and invasive cancer?	A **histological one**. Carcinoma-in-situ (CIS) implies that the cancer is **confined by the basement membrane** of the ducts and lobules.
What types of CIS do you know of?	Ductal (DCIS) and lobular (LCIS) Ductal CIS is more common than lobular. High grade CIS carry a worse prognosis and 20–30% progress to an invasive cancer.
What are the main types of breast cancer?	All breast cancers arise from either the DCIS (90%) or LCIS (10%). **Ductal sub-types:** • Invasive non-specific duct carcinoma (85%) • Medullary carcinoma • Tubular carcinoma • Mucoid carcinoma • Papillary carcinoma • Paget's disease of the nipple. **Lobular sub-types:** • Invasive lobular carcinoma (10%).
What is Paget's disease of the nipple?	Breast cancer that may or may not be palpable clinically but is associated with a unilateral, bleeding, eczematous nipple.

What risk factors are associated with breast cancer?	1. Previous history of breast cancer
	2. Early menarche/late menopause
	3. Nulliparity (no pregnancies)
	4. Oral contraceptive pill
	5. Hormone replacement therapy
	6. Positive family history
	7. Breast feeding
	8. Alcohol
	9. Smoking.

What is the oestrogen window?

The period of time a woman is exposed to oestrogen. Oestrogen exposure is linked to ↑ incidence of breast cancer as many tumours have **oestrogen receptors (ER)**. Numbers 2–5 above are risk factors because of this.

What percentage of tumours are oestrogen dependent?

30% of all tumours are oestrogen dependent. 60% ER positive patients respond to hormone therapy (see below), compared to 10% ER negative patients.

So what are considered to be protective factors?

Factors which ↓ the oestrogen window:
1. Late menarche/early menopause
2. Multiparity (>1 pregnancy; pregnancy is an **oestrogen-free** period).

Is breast cancer hereditary?

Yes. A positive family history of breast cancer among first-degree relatives is significant because 5–10% breast cancers are inherited in an **autosomal dominant** manner with **limited penetrance**. These patients usually present at an earlier age and there may also be a family history of ovarian, colon and other cancers.

Which genes are implicated in the inheritance of breast cancer?	*BRCA 1* (chrm 17q 21) *BRCA 2* (chrm 13q 24) *p53* (chrm 17p). (Remember, **p** is for *petit* which means **short** in French; hence **short chromosomal arm.** The **long chromosomal arm** is denoted by **q**, only because it follows **p** alphabetically!)
How does breast cancer spread?	**Lymphatic:** majority move laterally to the axillary lymph nodes; a small proportion spread medially to the internal mammary nodes. **Bloodstream:** liver, lungs, bone and brain. **Transcoelomic:** both pleural and peritoneal seeding may occur in advanced disease.
What are the important points in the history?	1. Ask about the lump: how and when noticed; painful; recent changes; associated nipple changes. 2. Ask about risk factors (see above; a full gynaecological history is *mandatory*). 3. Ask about symptoms suggesting metastasis: • Jaundice (liver mets) • Back/limb pain (spinal/bony mets) • Headaches; mood changes; visual disturbances (brain mets) • SOB/haemoptysis (lung mets) • Weight loss (cancer cachexia).
What are the examination findings?	*General:* cachexia, jaundice *Breast: Inspection (done with hand on hips, then hands held above head):* obvious **mass** (causing breast asymmetry; fungating?); **skin** (puckered; reddened; pitted [*peau*

d'orange, ie orange-skin 2ry to infiltration of skin lymphatics by tumour]); **nipple** (eczematous lesion [Paget's disease]; discharge [bloody])
Palpation (done with patient lying flat and ipsilateral hand behind head): hard, **scirrhous** lump with ill-defined edges, attached to skin, nipple or underlying muscle, or all three?
Axilla: lymphadenopathy; feel for all groups (see anatomy section above)
Systemic: auscultate chest (lung involvement); palpate abdomen (feel for liver involvement); percuss spine (spinal involvement).

What are the investigations?

Triple assessment:
1. History/examination
2. USS/mammogram
3. FNAC.
In addition:

Blood investigations:
1. FBC: anaemia of chronic disease
2. LFTs: liver involvement; also ↑ALP in bony involvement; ↓albumin in cachexia
3. Bone profile: bony involvement (↑Ca).

Imaging:
1. CXR: lung involvement (obvious mets or pleural effusion)
2. Liver USS: liver mets
3. CT chest/abdomen: staging of cancer (lung, liver, lymph nodes).

Pathology:
1. FNAC (cells only, for cytology)
2. Trucut biopsy (core biopsy supplying tissue for histology)
3. Excision biopsy (lump removed for histology).

What ways are there of staging breast cancer?

TNM classification: takes into account the size of the **T**umour, degree of lymphadenopathy (**N**odes), and presence/absence of **M**etastases. **Manchester staging** (see Figure 43.1):

Figure 43.1 Manchester Classification of Breast Cancer

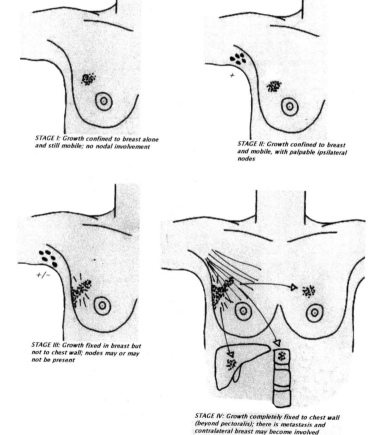

STAGE I: Growth confined to breast alone and still mobile; no nodal involvement

STAGE II: Growth confined to breast and mobile, with palpable ipsilateral nodes

STAGE III: Growth fixed in breast but not to chest wall; nodes may or may not be present

STAGE IV: Growth completely fixed to chest wall (beyond pectoralis); there is metastasis and contralateral breast may become involved

- **Stage 1** Growth is confined to the breast alone with no nodal involvement, however is still mobile.
- **Stage 2** As above, and there are palpable lymph nodes on the ipsilateral side
- **Stage 3** The tumour is fixed to the pectoralis muscle (but not the chest wall) and there may or may not be lymphadenopathy
- **Stage 4** There is complete fixation of the tumour to the chest wall. There are also distant mets and the contralateral breast may also be affected.

How can treatment of breast cancer be remembered?

Treat the breast, treat the axilla, treat the rest.

What are the treatment options in breast cancer?

Breast: wide local excision vs. mastectomy
Axillary nodes: clearance vs. radiotherapy
Systemic: several options: radiotherapy, chemotherapy, hormonal therapy (see below).

What is the role of surgery in treatment of breast cancer?

Surgery does not decrease mortality. Its main aim is to control local disease and prevent progression.
Surgery is not the only option for breast cancer patients, nor is it suitable for everyone but if performed it is usually curative in nature.

What factors should be taken into account before deciding on surgery?

These include:
1. The patient's age
2. Their general medical state and fitness for surgery
3. The stage of disease
4. The patient's own wishes.

What surgical options are there?

Wide local excision: preferred option for small, well-localised tumours and should be followed by radiotherapy of the remaining breast post-operatively.

Mastectomy: done in the following situations:

- Large tumours (>3.5 cm)
- Central tumours ie involving the nipple
- Ill-defined tumours
- Multiple lesions
- Patient's choice.

What types of mastectomy do you know of?

Radical mastectomy (Halsted procedure):

The following are removed:

- Breast (including nipple)
- Surrounding skin and fascia
- Pectoralis major (sternal part) and minor
- Costocoracoid membrane
- Axillary fat, fascia and nodes.

Rarely used.

Modified radical mastectomy (Patey procedure): as above, but pectoralis major is preserved.

Simple mastectomy: only the breast is removed. The axilla is not cleared. Most commonly used in conjunction with axillary node sampling or sentinel node biopsy.

What are the complications of mastectomy?

Early:

Wound infection

Wound haematoma

Damage to the intercostobrachial nerve (loss of sensation in the axilla; occurs during axillary surgery).

Late:
Lymphoedema of the upper limb (2ry to axillary clearance of radiotherapy)
Breast seroma
Frozen shoulder.

What is the importance of staging the axilla?

In the absence of distant metastases, the presence or absence of axillary lymph node involvement provides the best indicator of prognosis.

How is this done?

Either by **axillary sampling** or **sentinel node biopsy**.
Axillary sampling: 4 lymph nodes are chosen and depending on if they are affected, the decision is made whether the patient requires total axillary clearance or post-operative radiotherapy.
Sentinel node biopsy: The sentinel node is the first node that a section of the breast drains to. If this is sampled and cleared of tumour then it is highly unlikely other nodes would be affected. This is done by injecting a dye containing a radioisotope into the tumour, and identifying the first axillary node it spreads to (the sentinel node) by use of a Geiger counter.

What is axillary clearance?

This is removal of the axillary lymph nodes that the cancer is believed to have spread to based on sampling. Clearance can be level I, II or III (see anatomy above).

What nerves are at risk of injury in axillary clearance?

1. Long thoracic n. (of Bell): serratus anterior; damage causes winging of the scapula.
2. Thoracodorsal n.: latissimus dorsi

3. Medial pectoral n.: pectoralis major and minor
4. Lateral pectoral n.: pectoralis major and minor
5. Intercostobrachial n.: sensory supply to axilla.

What is the role of systemic therapy?

This can be either **adjuvant** or **neo-adjuvant**.

Radiotherapy:

- Post-operatively to improve prognosis: given to the **breast** if a wide local excision is performed; given to the **axilla** if axillary sampling or sentinel node biopsy is done and cancer is detected. (*No radiotherapy* to breast if mastectomy is done; *no radiotherapy* to axilla if clearance is done [risk of arm lymphoedema])
- Palliative for pain control in advanced disease.

Chemotherapy: mainly CMF (cyclophosphamide, methotrexate, 5-fluorouracil)

- Positive axillary nodes
- Recurrent disease
- Large tumours
- High grade tumours
- All post-menopausal women.

Hormonal therapy: oestrogen receptor antagonists or SERM (selective oestrogen receptor modulators) (1st line, eg tamoxifen; see below), aromatase inhibitors (2nd line, eg anastrazole), luteinising hormone releasing hormone (LHRH) antagonists (also 2nd line, eg goserelin) and progesterone (3rd line).

What is tamoxifen?	A partial agonist of oestrogen at its receptor.
When is it used?	To treat advanced disease, especially in those with ER positive tumours. (In ER negative patients, the risks of hormonal therapy should be considered and chemotherapy might be an alternative.) Can only be used for a maximum of 5 years. Long-term use is associated with an increased risk of developing **endometrial cancer**.
Apart from lymph node involvement, how can prognosis be assessed?	**Nottingham prognostic index:** (0.2 $\times$ tumour size in cm) + lymph node stage + tumour histological grade
What is the long term prognosis for breast cancer patients?	5-year survival rate for stage 1 tumours is 80%, and falls as stage increases. In addition to the stage of disease, prognosis depends on its histological grade ie a high grade tumour has a worse prognosis.
What is the follow-up post-op?	3-monthly for 1 year (plus adjuvant therapy), 6-monthly for 4 years, then yearly for 5 years. At these visits, evidence for distal recurrence of disease is sought.
What about the breasts?	If **conservation surgery** has been done (eg lumpectomy), the rest of the affected breast should undergo yearly mammography. In all post-op women, the contralateral breast can undergo mammography every 2 years.

How is breast cancer screened?

In women 40 years and over, annual clinical examination and 2-view mammography. In women aged 20–39, clinical examination every 3 years supplemented with monthly self-examination.

Figure 43.2 An algorithm for the management of a palpable breast mass

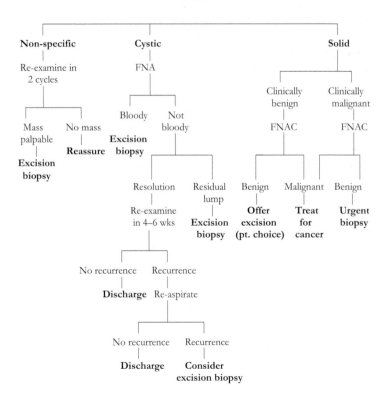

Palpable breast mass

Triple Assessment:
History / Examination
Imaging: <30 = USS; >30 = USS + mammogram
FNAC

Non-specific
Re-examine in 2 cycles

Mass palpable
Excision biopsy

No mass
Reassure

Cystic
FNA

Bloody
Excision biopsy

Not bloody

Resolution
Re-examine in 4–6 wks

No recurrence
Discharge

Recurrence
Re-aspirate

No recurrence
Discharge

Recurrence
Consider excision biopsy

Residual lump
Excision biopsy

Solid

Clinically benign
FNAC

Benign
Offer excision (pt. choice)

Malignant
Treat for cancer

Clinically malignant
FNAC

Benign
Urgent biopsy

CHAPTER 44: RENAL CARCINOMA

What types of kidney cancer do you know of?

Renal cell carcinoma (RCC)
Transitional cell carcinoma (TCC)
These 2 make up the majority of renal cancers.

Which one is more common?

RCC by far: 90%
TCC occurs in the transitional cell-lined areas of the kidney such as the renal pelvis, but is the most common cancer of the bladder (see Chapter 45).

When people speak of kidney cancer, what is understood unless otherwise stated?

RCC!

What is RCC also known as?

Grawitz tumour (pronounced **gra**-*vitz*).

Where does RCC arise from?

Proximal tubular cells in the renal cortex which then grow outwards to compress the renal parenchymal tissue. This compressed renal parenchymal tissue together with fibrous tissue constitutes the **pseudocapsule**.

What does the tumour look like?

High lipid content gives it a yellow to orange appearance macroscopically.

Who gets RCC?

Occurs most commonly in 5th to 6th decade M:F = 2:1. The incidence of RCC is higher in black men as compare to other races.

What is its aetiology?

The cause of RCC is unknown. Risk factors include:
1. Cigarette smoking
2. Von Hippel–Lindau disease
3. Horse shoe kidney
4. Adult polycystic kidney disease
5. Acquired cystic disease of kidneys.

Which chromosome is affected in RCC?	Chromosome 3.
How does RCC present?	**Classic triad:** 1. Haematuria (micro- or macroscopic) 2. Loin pain 3. Flank mass.
How often does this classical presentation occur?	Only 10% of the time!
So what is the most common presentation?	Micro- or macroscopic haematuria alone (60%). Some patients may present incidentally (having scans for other reasons), or with metastatic disease.
What is RCC famous for?	Paraneoplastic syndromes (10–40% of patients with RCC).
What is a paraneoplastic syndrome?	The collective signs and symptoms caused by a substance emanating from a tumour or in reaction to a tumour. A paraneoplastic syndrome is not produced by the primary tumour itself or by its metastases, nor is it caused by compression, infection, nutritional deficiency, or treatment of the tumour.

What paraneoplastic syndromes are associated with RCC?	1. Erythrocytosis: ↑erythropoietin (EPO) production from the juxtaglomerular apparatus (JGA)
	2. Hypercalcaemia: ↑ parathyroid hormone related peptide (PTHrP) production by the tumour
	3. Hypertension: ↑ renin from JGA
	4. Non-metastatic hepatic dysfunction: a syndrome of:
	  a. Hepatosplenomegaly
	  b. ↑ ALP
	  c. ↑ serum haptoglobin
	  d. ↑ prothrombin (bleeding) time
	(syn. **Stauffer's syndrome**).

What are the common sites for metastasis?

Renal carcinoma generally metastasises to **lungs**. Bone and liver metastasis can also occur.

What facilitates metastasis to the lungs?

Extension of tumour along renal vein and into the IVC.

What are the investigations performed for RCC?

Blood investigations:
1. FBC: anaemia 2ry to haematuria
2. U&Es: may be deranged in extensive renal involvement
3. LFTs: deranged in Stauffer's syndrome
4. Bone profile: hypercalcaemia may be present
5. Clotting: deranged in Stauffer's syndrome.

Imaging:
1. **CXR:** lung mets
2. **USS kidneys:** shows tumour and IVC extension
3. **CT abdomen and pelvis:** for staging of the disease (also CT chest if CXR equivocal)
4. **Bone scan:** for bone metastasis.

How would you stage RCC?

TNM staging system is used for deciding management for RCC.

T0: no evidence of primary tumour
T1: <7 cm confined to kidney
T2: >7 cm but confined to kidney
T3: tumour extends into adrenal gland or perinephric fat or renal vein or inferior vena cava but not extending beyond Gerota's fascia
T4: tumour extending beyond Gerota's fascia
N0: no lymph node involvement
N1: single node 2 cm or less

N2: more than one regional node involved

M0: no distant metastasis

M1: distant metastasis.

What is Gerota's fascia?
The connective tissue capsule of the kidney.

What are the treatment options?
Depends on the stage of the disease. In general:

Localised disease:
1. **Radical nephrectomy:** for patients with a normal contralateral kidney.
2. **Partial nephrectomy:** is used in the following patients :
   a. Single kidney
   b. Bilateral tumours
   c. Impaired contralateral kidney function
   d. Tumour <4 cm
   (syn. **nephron-sparing surgery**).

Involvement of IVC: these patients benefit from nephrectomy and removal of tumour thrombus from IVC. 50–60% 5-year survival has been reported in these patients.

Metastatic disease: surgical excision of a solitary resectable metastatic lesion with nephrectomy is warranted. **Adjuvant therapeutic modalities** are:
a. **Chemotherapy:** not very effective in metastatic disease.
b. **Immunotherapy:** α-interferon and interleukin-2 have recently shown good results in trials.
c. **Radiotherapy:** can be used for bone metastasis.

What is the prognosis?
Again, depends on the stage: Overall, 5-year survival ranges from 60 to 82% for small RCC confined to the

kidney. For RCC that extends into major veins, adrenal glands, or perinephric tissue, but not beyond Gerota's fascia, the 5-year survival averages 50%.

CHAPTER 45: BLADDER CARCINOMA

What is the incidence of bladder cancer?

45/100,000. M:F = 3:1.

Where is the most common place for transitional cell carcinoma (TCC) to arise?

90% of transitional cell carcinomas are found in the bladder.

Where else can TCC be found?

Transitional epithelium lines the urinary tract from the collecting systems in the kidneys to the proximal urethra. TCC can occur at any point.

Apart from TCC, what other types of bladder cancer are there?

The majority (>90%) of bladder cancers are **transitional cell**. Others include:
1. Squamous cell carcinoma (SCC)
2. Adenocarcinoma (*rare!*).

When people speak of bladder cancer, what type is understood unless otherwise stated?

TCC!

What are the risk factors?

TCC:
1. Smoking
2. History of bladder diverticulae
3. Schistosomiasis
4. Aromatic hydrocarbons used in the rubber and dye industries.

SCC: pts. more likely to have a history of chronic irritation or inflammation eg stones or schistosomiasis causing metaplasia.

How does bladder cancer present?

80% of patients present with painless haematuria as the only symptom, most commonly at the end of micturition. There may also be:
- Irritative signs (frequency, urgency)
- CRF (if ureteric orifices become obstructed by cancer causing urinary outflow blockage).

Where does bladder cancer spread to?

Directly to urethra, prostate, colon, rectum, uterus and vagina.
Lymphatics: para-aortic and iliac nodes
Blood-borne: liver and lungs (late).

What are the investigations?

A haematuria screen (see Chapter 26). Also:
Once bladder cancer is suspected, staging of disease is important:
- USS/CT-guided biopsy
- CXR: chest mets
- CT thorax/abdomen: mets and lymph node involvement
- Bone scan: bony mets.

What is the staging system for bladder cancer (TCC)?

Bladder cancers are staged according to the TNM System. **T**umour is as follows:
T1 superficial to the bladder muscle ie confined to the mucosa/submucosa
T2 involving the superficial muscle
T3 involvement of deep muscle or perivesical fat
T4 invasion of adjacent structures.

What is the treatment?

Treatment depends on the stage of the tumour:
T1 transurethral resection of the bladder tumour (TURBT) or intravesical chemotherapy with either mitomycin or BCG (Bacille Calmette–Guérin).
T2/T3 **radical cystectomy** with ileal conduit for younger patients who are fit for surgery, whereas radiotherapy may be more suitable for older patients
T4 palliative radiotherapy.

What is the prognosis?

The higher the stage of the cancer, the poorer the prognosis. However overall 1/3 of bladder cancer patients survive 5 years. 5-year survival falls from 90% to 45% once there is deep muscle involvement.

CHAPTER 46: PROSTATIC CARCINOMA

What is the prevalence of prostate cancer?

It is the most common cancer diagnosed and 2nd most common cause of cancer deaths in males. Its prevalence increases with age. About 30% of males above 50 years have histological evidence of prostate carcinoma.

What is its aetiology?

Various risk factors have been identified:
1. Advanced age
2. Afro-Caribbean ethnic origin
3. Family history
4. Increased fat diet
5. Smoking.

What is the pathology?

More than 90% are adenocarcinomas. Rare types can be transitional cell carcinoma and sarcomas.

Which prostatic zone typically forms cancer?

Prostate carcinomas typically form in peripheral zone (70%). 20% arise in transitional zone and 10% in central zone.

What are its main symptoms?

Mainly asymptomatic in majority of patients because it involves the **peripheral zone** of the prostate (hence no urethral obstruction). In these patients it is diagnosed as an incidental finding on histology of TURP chips, or from a high PSA level (see below). Symptoms generally indicate a **locally advanced** or **metastatic** disease.

Involvement of urethra or bladder neck can lead to obstructive and irritative symptoms (see Chapter 34c). Bony metastasis (mainly to lumbar spine) can lead to pain and signs of nerve compression.

What are the classical findings of prostate cancer on DRE?

Enlarged (>20 g) hard, craggy prostate with no palpable median sulcus, a tethered overlying rectovesical fascia (of Denonvilliers). (NB findings may reveal a singular nodule only.)

What are the investigations?

Blood investigations:
1. Prostate specific antigen (PSA): usually raised
2. LFTs: ALP may be raised in bony mets.

Imaging:
1. Transrectal USS (TRUS): biopsy can be performed at the same time (TRUS biopsy)
2. CT and MRI (for staging the disease: local invasion and metastatic spread)
3. Bone scan (for bone metastasis).

What is PSA?

PSA is an enzyme normally secreted by prostate epithelium.

What are causes for high PSA?

A high PSA is **not specific** to carcinoma. It can be elevated in:
- BPH
- UTIs
- Prostatitis
- Urethral instrumentation
- Urine retention.

However, a high PSA should warrant further investigation, such as TRUS biopsy of the prostate.

What is Gleason grading?

Gleason is the most commonly used grading system for prostate carcinoma. This grading is based on the histological **glandular architectural pattern**. More than 1 pattern usually exists. The most commonly occurring pattern is known as the 1ry grade and the 2nd commonest is known as the 2ry grade. Gleason grading scores the 1ry and 2ry grades from 1 to 5. The more poorly differentiated the grade, the higher the grading score.

Gleason score is achieved by adding the grading scores of the 1ry and 2ry grades together eg if a patient's tumour has a 1ry grade of Gleason 4 and a 2ry grade of Gleason 2, the Gleason score will be $4+2$ (6). High Gleason scores indicate more aggressive disease.

What are the clinical stages of prostate carcinoma?

Prostate carcinoma is staged according to TNM System. T means tumour size, N for lymph node and M for distant metastasis (generally bones).

Tx Cannot be assessed

T0 No evidence of primary tumour

Tis Carcinoma-in-situ (prostatic intraepithelial neoplasia; PIN)

T1 No clinical evidence (DRE and imaging normal); TURP chips show carcinoma

T2 Confined to prostate

T3 Extracapsular extension

T4 Fixed tumour involving other pelvic structures like rectum and bladder neck

What are the commonest sites for metastasis?

Prostate carcinoma generally metastasises to bones with lumbar spine the commonest site. Other sites are the femur, pelvis, thoracic spine, and ribs.

What is the special feature of bony metastasis in prostate carcinoma?

Prostatic bony metastases are typically osteoblastic and thus appear **sclerotic** on X-rays as compared to **lytic** in other types of bony metastasis.

What are the treatment options?	Treatment options available are: **Localised disease:** • **Watchful waiting:** patients who have low grade disease and life expectancy less than 10 years. • **Radical prostatectomy**: young, fit patients with localised disease. • **Radiotherapy:** patients who are surgically high risk (performed as **brachytherapy**; radioactive beads are placed in the prostate at specifically mapped points. As they decay, they emit radioactivity which destroys cancer cells). **Locally advanced carcinoma:** this is generally treated with neoadjuvant hormone therapy followed by radiotherapy. Stage T3 tumours are generally included in this category. **Metastatic disease:** • Hormone therapy • Radiotherapy can be used in bone metastasis for pain relief.
What is the aim of hormone therapy?	To block the action of testosterone, as prostate cancer is **testosterone-dependent**.
What type of hormone therapy is used in prostate cancer?	Drugs (**chemical castration**) 1. **LHRH analogues** eg goserelin, buserelin 2. **Anti-androgens** eg flutamide. Surgery: removal of the testicles, and hence the source of testosterone (bilateral orchidectomy or **surgical castration**).
How do they work?	**LHRH analogues** block the pituitary by a feedback mechanism, and thus decrease secretion of testosterone leading to atrophy of tumour cells. **Anti-androgens** block the effect of androgens on target tissues by occupying the receptors.

What is complete androgen blockade?

Testosterone is produced by the Leydig cells in the testes but small amount of androgens are also produced by the adrenals. LHRH analogues only control the testicular androgens. If an anti-androgen and an LHRH analogue are used in combination, then complete androgen blockade is achieved as target tissues are also blocked.

CHAPTER 47: TESTICULAR, PENILE AND SCROTAL CARCINOMA

TESTICULAR CARCINOMA

What types of testicular cancers do you know?	**Germ cell tumours (GCT)** and **non-germ cell tumours**. **Germ cell tumours (95%):** Seminomas (45%) Non-seminomatous germ cell tumours (NSGCT; 50%) • Mixed cell type (most common; 50%) • Teratoma • Embryonal cell tumour • Choriocarcinoma (rare) • Yolk sac tumours (most common pre-pubertal tumours). **Non-germinal tumours (5%):** • Leydig cell tumour • Sertoli cell tumour. These are all **primary** tumours. Cancers may also be **secondary**, such as lymphoma and leukaemia.
What is treatment based on?	Whether the tumour is a seminoma or a NSGCT (the various NSGCT subtypes are nice to know, but do not alter the treatment given!)
What is testicular cancer known as?	A cancer of young men. It is the most common solid malignancy of males aged 18–35, but represents only 1% of *all* cancers in males of all ages.
What are risk factors for developing testicular cancer?	1. History of contralateral testicular cancer 2. Cryptorchidism (undescended testes) 3. Ectopic testes 4. Family history 5. Testicular dysgenesis

6. Oestradiol exposure *in utero*
7. Chemical carcinogens (eg dinitrotoluene)
8. Trauma
9. Orchitis (especially mumps).

How does it spread?

Seminomas: lymphatic spread to para-aortic nodes (and *not* to the inguinal nodes!)
Teratomas: also spread via lymphatics, but can undergo blood-borne spread to liver, lung, bone, and brain as well.

Why do seminomas spread to the para-aortic nodes first?

The para-aortic nodes drain the testes of lymph (remember, *not* the inguinal nodes which drain the scrotum; this is a famous trick question!). Keep in mind that the testes were once **intra-abdominal structures** before their descent. Their lymph nodes didn't follow them.

How does it present?

Usually as a painless lump (but *may* be painful) discovered either on self-examination, or at a routine check-up.
β-HCG-producing tumours may cause gynaecomastia, the only presenting complaint.

What are the clinical findings?

Genitals: firm to hard immobile mass on testicle, usually non-tender, not transilluminable. There may be a non-traumatic haematocele (see Chapter 34d). Usually *no palpable inguinal nodes* (see above). **Examine other testicle!**
General: examine back (tenderness), lungs (effusion) and abdomen (hepatomegaly): all site of metastases. Look for gynaecomastia and jaundice (liver mets). Palpate

lymph nodes which drain the para-aortic nodes for signs of distal spread (eg Virchow's nodes in the supraclavicular fossa).

What are the investigations?

Blood investigations:
- Tumour markers (see Table 47.1)
- FBC: anaemia if metastatic disease
- LFTs: raised in liver mets
- LDH: used to monitor response to therapy and as a prognostic factor
- U&Es: may be deranged in lymphatic spread (see below).

Imaging:
- **CXR:** pleural effusion and obvious mets
- **Scrotal USS:** confirms the suspicion of what is mainly a clinical diagnosis
- **CT scan:** full body scan for staging of the tumour
- **IVU:** to assess the ureters (see below).

Table 47.1

	α-fetoprotein (AFP)	β-HCG
Seminoma	No	Yes
Teratoma	Yes	No
Embryonal cell	Yes	No
Choriocarcinoma	No	Yes
Yolk sac	Yes	No

What are the chances of these tumour markers being present?

Tumour markers only present in 8% of seminomas and 60% of NSGCTs.

How may testicular cancer cause deranged renal function?

More common in seminomas which spread to the retroperitoneal para-aortic lymph nodes. The ureters are also retroperitoneal. Grossly enlarged lymph nodes may compress the ureter(s).

How is testicular cancer staged?

With the **Royal Marsden Staging System:**

I Disease confined to testis; no evidence of metastases

    Is Stage I on surveillance

    Im Stage I on CT but marker positive.

II Infra-diaphragmatic lymph node involvement

    IIA Lymph nodes < 2 cm

    IIB Lymph nodes 2–5 cm

    IIC Lymph nodes >5 cm

III Supra-diaphragmatic lymph node involvement.

    IIIA,B,C As with III but with abdominal disease (lymph node sizes as in II).

IV Extra lymphatic mets

    L1 < 3 lung mets

    L2 > 3 lung mets

    L3 > 3 lung mets, 1 or more being > 2 cm

    H+ Hepatic involvement

    Br+ Brain involvement

    M+ Mediastinum involvement

    N+ Neck nodal involvement.

(TNM classification also used.)

What is the management?

Orchidectomy (surgical removal of the testicle) in all patients.

How is this performed?

Via an **inguinal incision**, the diseased testicle is pulled out and excised with its spermatic cord (known as the **inguinal approach**).

Why not use a scrotal approach?

For fear of seeding the scrotum with cancer cells which may then spread to the inguinal nodes (*here* the

	inguinal nodes are important!) and then on to the iliac nodes.
What about adjuvant therapy?	**Seminoma:** these tumours are highly treatable and **radiosensitive**. Stages I and II get ipsilateral radiotherapy to the nodes *or* undergo **surveillance** (disease is followed up closely following orchidectomy, looking for progression). Stage IIC and above get **platinum-based chemotherapy** (cisplatin). **NSGCT:** these tumours are **radio-*in*sensitive**. Stage I treated with surveillance only following orchidectomy (retroperitoneal lymph node dissection [RPLND] is performed in the USA). In Stage I relapses and metastatic disease (ie stage II and above), **BEP** (**b**leomycin, **e**toposide, cis**p**latin) is given.
What is the prognosis?	Good for seminomas (stage I = 95% survival rate at 5 years); less good for NSGCTs (stage I = 86% at 5 years).

PENILE CARCINOMA

What are the risk factors for penile cancer?	1. Lack of circumcision 2. Smegma: accumulation of secretions from the foreskin glands (Tyson's glands) which collect under the foreskin giving a cheesy appearance (colloquially known as 'cheese') 3. Phimosis (smegma accumulation) 4. Poor hygiene (also connected to smegma accumulation) 5. Low socio-economic bracket 6. Viruses: HPV 16 & 18 (cause genital warts)

7. Pre-malignant conditions of the penis (carcinoma-in-situ [CIS]):
   a. Erythroplasia of Queyrat (E of Q; Bowen's disease of the penis)
   b. Bowenoid papulosis
   c. Balanitis xerotica obliterans (BXO)
   d. Leucoplakia
   e. Buschke–Lowenstein giant condyloma.

Who have almost 0% chance of developing penile cancer?

Jewish men, due to circumcision at birth (Muslims also have very low incidence for similar reasons, but a slightly higher incidence than Jews as they are circumcised later).

What is the most common type of penile cancer?

Squamous cell carcinoma.

Which part of the penis is most commonly affected?

The glans (48%) or prepuce (foreskin; 21%).

How does it present?

As either a fungating or ulcerating lesion (usually painless). There may be associated bleeding.

What nodes become affected during spread?

Inguinal nodes first, then on to iliac nodes.

When does spread occur?

Late. Limited by Buck's fascia (the deep fascia of the penis).

What are the investigations?

1. Biopsy of the lesion
2. CXR (r/o mets)
3. CT abdomen and pelvis (staging)
4. 1% toluidine + 1% acetic acid detects CIS.

What is the treatment?

Divided into treatment of the penis and of the inguinal nodes.
Penis:
CIS: For preputial lesions, circumcision may be enough;

otherwise, excision biopsy. Alternatives include:

- Topical chemotherapy (5-fluorouracil)
- NdYAG or CO_2 laser
- Radiotherapy.

Carcinoma: partial or full penile amputation (penectomy).

Inguinal nodes: if clinically swollen, give a course of antibiotics and observe to see if swelling settles. If not, block dissection of the lymph nodes +/– radiotherapy if extensive.

Define the following.

E of Q: a chronic pre-cancerous condition presenting with circumscribed **red velvety lesion** at the mucocutaneous junction of the mouth, vulva, penis, or prepuce.

Bowen's disease: squamous cell carcinoma *in situ* with a potential for significant lateral spread. When it occurs on the penis, it is known as E of Q.

Bowenoid papulosis: a rare, sexually transmitted disorder thought to be caused by HPV type 16 and characterised by lesions that are reddish brown or violet in colour, small, solid, raised, and sometimes velvety.

Balanitis xerotica obliterans (BXO): a chronic, progressive, sclerosing inflammatory dermatosis of unclear aetiology. Most reported cases (83%) involve the genitalia. May present as mild, nonspecific erythema or mild hypopigmentation. (Syn. **genital lichen sclerosis**.)

Leucoplakia: a white patch or plaque that cannot be rubbed off, cannot be characterised clinically or histologically as any other condition, and is not associated with any physical or chemical causative agent. Mainly occurs in the mouth (where tobacco, alcohol and chronic irritation from ill-fitting dentures are seen as possibly causative), but rarely occurs on the genitals, where the cause is unknown.

Buschke–Lowenstein giant condyloma (GCBL): a slow-growing, locally destructive verrucous lesion, possibly of viral aetiology, that typically appears on the penis (usually glans) but may occur elsewhere in the anogenital region. Low metastatic potential.

SCROTAL CARCINOMA

What type of cancer is it?	Squamous cell carcinoma.
How common is it?	No longer common.
Who was most prone to getting it?	Chimney sweeps who climbed up chimneys to clean them. The soot was carcinogenic. (This is a favourite question!)
How does it present?	As a painless, ulcerating scrotal lesion which may or may not bleed.
Where does it spread to?	The inguinal nodes and then on to the iliac nodes.
How is a diagnosis made?	Clinical suspicion and biopsy.
What is the management?	Excision of the lesion and management of affected nodes (as with penile cancer; see above).

CHAPTER 48: ENDOCRINE CARCINOMA: THYROID, PARATHYROID, AND ADRENALS

THYROID CARCINOMA

What types do you know of?

1. Papillary (most common; 80%)
2. Follicular (10%)
3. Medullary
4. Anaplastic
5. Lymphoma.

What are papillary, follicular and medullary cancers also known as?

Differentiated thyroid cancers.

What are the predisposing factors of thyroid cancer?

mnemonic: **CRISP**
Chronic lymphocytic thyroiditis (Hashimoto's, a risk factor for lymphoma)
Relatives with thyroid cancer (genetics)
Ionising radiation
Solitary thyroid nodule
Prolonged stimulation by raised TSH.

Can you compare them?

See Table 48.1

Table 48.1

	Papillary	**Follicular**	**Medullary**	**Anaplastic**
Incidence	All age groups, but peak at 40–49 years	50–59 years	50–59 years	Elderly
	F:M = 3:1 in all variants			
Histological features	Cells containing **psammoma bodies** and clear, ground-glass nuclei (**orphan Annie** nuclei)	An **absence** of psammoma bodies; carcinoma and adenoma are **indistinguishable** on FNAC	Arise from calcitonin-secreting **parafollicular C cells**	No characteristic architecture and does not resemble normal thyroid tissue

Table 48.1 (continued)

	Papillary	Follicular	Medullary	Anaplastic
Presentation	Solitary thyroid lump	Solitary thyroid lump	May be solitary, or multiple if occurring as part of **MEN IIa or IIb** (see Chapter 33d)	Aggressive tumour with early spread to surrounding structures, including trachea, oesophagus, recurrent laryngeal nerve
Spread	Mainly lymphatic to regional lymph nodes (60%) *mnemonic:* papillar**y** ends in **y** and **y** stands for **y**ellow which is the colour of lymph	Mainly haematogenous to bone and lung (20–30%) *mnemonic:* follicula**r** ends in **r** and **r** stands for **r**ed which is the colour of blood	Lymphatic spread in 25% of cases	Local, lymphatic and haematogenous
Investigations	**Blood investigations:** thyroid function tests **Imaging:** 1. **CXR:** r/o retrosternal spread and lung mets 2. **USS neck:** measures tumour size, r/o multinodular goitre and contralateral disease 3. **CT neck:** staging of cancer (size, nodal involvement, and invasion) 4. **Scintigraphy:** not commonly used now; shows a **cold nodule** on scan (non-active) **FNAC:** gives a cytological diagnosis which confirms or dispels suspicion. Follicular carcinoma and adenoma cannot be distinguished on FNAC, so *a follicular reading is taken as cancer until proven otherwise.*			
Prognosis	Excellent with a 90% long-term survival rate	Excellent; mean survival rate at 10 years is 60%	Good; may be aggressive if associated with MEN, however, with poorer prognosis	Poor; 5-year survival rate is <10%

What are psammoma bodies?

Structure found in some benign or malignant tumour cells. They look like hardened concentric rings when viewed under a microscope. They can be a sign of chronic inflammation.

What factors make a patient with differentiated thyroid cancer high or low risk?

High risk:
1. Females >45 years
2. Being male
3. All patients <16 years

Low risk: females <45 years.

What factors make the *tumour* high or low risk?

High risk:
1. Tumour >1 cm
2. Multifocal tumours
3. Metastasis.

Low risk:
1. Papillary carcinoma <1 cm
2. Minimally invasive follicular carcinoma <1 cm.

What is the management of differentiated thyroid cancer?

Controversial! Differs from centre to centre.

Check local policy, but *in general*:

Papillary and follicular cancers:
Low-risk patient and low-risk tumour: lobectomy
Low-risk patient and high-risk tumour: lobectomy or total thyroidectomy
High-risk patient with low-risk tumour: lobectomy or total thyroidectomy
High-risk patient with high-risk tumour: total thyroidectomy.
Medullary cancers: total thyroidectomy.

Neck dissection of the lymph nodes is performed if there is nodal involvement.

What about adjuvant therapy?	**Radioiodine** is given to detect and ablate all residual thyroid tissue and metastases. It is given until there is no more take-up detectable. This is only effective in **papillary** and **follicular** types. **Radiotherapy:** external beam radiotherapy is reserved for unresectable disease and disease non-responsive to radioiodine. Used in all types.
What must be done if adjuvant therapy is to be considered?	Total thyroidectomy (either at 1st operation or as a completion of a lobectomy).
Why?	If a lobe is left in situ, it will take up most or all of the radioiodine, leaving little for metastatic disease.
What should the patient be placed on following these modalities?	Thyroxine for resultant hypothyroidism.
How is anaplastic cancer treated?	Curative surgery and radiotherapy have no role. Surgery is purely palliative (eg isthmectomy for relief of tracheal compression). Palliative radiotherapy can be given to cause some regression, but re-growth is common.
What is the most common type of lymphoma affecting the thyroid?	High-grade B-cell non-Hodgkin's lymphoma.
What are the investigations?	As for the other types (see Table 48.1), but for lymphoma as well (see Chapter 50).
What is the management?	Treatment of lymphoma (see Chapter 50), though surgery can sometimes be done to debulk large tumours.

What is the management of a palpable solitary thyroid nodule?   See Figure 48.1.

Figure 48.1 Management of palpable solitary thyroid nodule

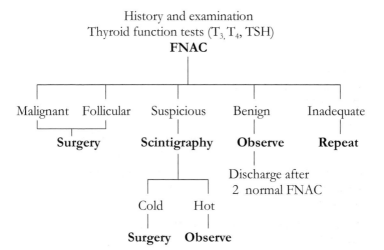

Palpable solitary thyroid nodule

History and examination
Thyroid function tests (T_3, T_4, TSH)
FNAC

Malignant   Follicular   Suspicious   Benign   Inadequate
Surgery   **Scintigraphy**   **Observe**   **Repeat**

Discharge after
2 normal FNAC

Cold   Hot
Surgery   **Observe**

PARATHYROID CARCINOMA

How common is it?	*Rare.*
What causes it?	Unknown.
What does it cause?	Hyperparathyroidism (see Chapter 33b).
How many patients with hyperparathyroidism have parathyroid cancer?	1%.
Who gets it?	M:F = 1:1; no age peak, but patients usually over 30 years old.

How does it present?	Usually incidentally during neck surgery for other reasons, or on histology of the thyroid gland with an incidentally included parathyroid gland. If it presents clinically, it may present as a **palpable** parathyroid gland, or as symptoms of hypercalcaemia ('bones, groans, stones, and abdominal moans').
What are the investigations?	**Blood investigations:** 1. Bone profile: extremely high Ca^{2+} levels (>3.0 mmol/L) 2. PTH: raised. **Imaging:** CT neck may show tumour.
How many glands are usually involved?	One.
How does it spread?	To lymph nodes (30%).
What is the management?	Wide local excision together with ipsilateral thyroid lobe and regional lymph nodes.
What about adjuvant therapy?	Radiotherapy if histology shows that the resection margins of the specimen are not clear of tumour. Chemotherapy is ineffective.
What is the prognosis?	50% survival rate at 5 years (poor).
What is death usually due to?	The metabolic consequences of hypercalcaemia.

ADRENAL CARCINOMA

What is the most common type?	Adenocarcinoma.
What part is usually involved?	The cortex.
How common is it?	*Rare.*

Who gets it?	F:M = 3:1; males get it older and have worse prognosis; females get it younger and usually have associated endocrine problems. Incidence is **bimodal** (2 peaks): kids less than 10, and then in mid-40s.
What causes it?	Unknown.
What is its main differential?	**Incidentaloma:** a benign, non-functional tumour of the adrenal gland, found on scans for other indications, and rarely requiring excision.
How are they broadly divided?	Into **functional** and **non-functional**. Functional type is associated with endocrine symptoms.
How does it present?	Usually late as metastatic disease. Non-functional cancer presents as a **flank mass**. Functional disease presents as an endocrine abnormality.
Which endocrine abnormality?	1. Cushing's syndrome (most common) 2. Conn's syndrome 3. Virilisation in girls 4. Precocious puberty or feminisation in boys (rare).
Name some syndromes it is associated with	1. Li–Fraumeni syndrome 2. FAP coli 3. Gardner's syndrome 4. Turcot's syndrome 5. Cowden syndrome 6. MEN I syndrome.
What are the investigations?	**Blood investigations:** these include screening tests for hormone excesses and possible syndromes (see Chapter 33c).

Special tests: based on suspected endocrine disorder (eg dexamethasone suppression test)
Imaging: CT/MRI scan of abdomen.

What is the management?

Surgical excision, chemotherapy (mitotane) for metastatic disease, and control of endocrine abnormalities if present.

CHAPTER 49: SKIN CANCER

What is the skin's claim to fame?

Largest organ in the body!

What are the levels of skin?

Epidermis: contains the **melanocytes**
Dermis: (mesenchymal)
Subcutaneous fat.

What are the layers of the epidermis?

mnemonic: **C**hicks **L**ove **G**ood **S**un **B**lock
Stratum **C**orneum
Stratum **L**ucidum
Stratum **G**ranulosum
Stratum **S**pinosum
Stratum **B**asale.

What is the dermis made up of?

Collagen, elastic fibres, and fat which support blood vessels, lymphatics and nerves.

What are melanocytes?

Skin cells of neuroectodermal origin which produce and contain **melanin**, the pigment responsible for skin colour.

What is a mole?

A cluster of melanocytes.

What is another name for a mole?

A **naevus**.

How do you categorise skin tumours?

In 2 ways: benign or malignant, or based on levels of skin involved.

Name some benign skin tumours.

Basal cell papilloma
Squamous cell papilloma
Keratoacanthoma.

Name some malignant skin tumours?

Basal cell carcinoma (BCC)
Squamous cell carcinoma (SCC)
Malignant melanoma (MM)
Kaposi's sarcoma.

What are the causes of skin cancer?

1. Sunlight
2. Topical carcinogens eg tar, rubber, dyes

3. Skin contaminants
4. Radiation eg X-rays
5. Genetic/congenital eg albinism
6. Viruses eg HPV.

What are the categories of normal skin?

Chalk white: burns easily and never tans
Fair: difficult to tan
Fair: easy to tan
Brown
Black.

Who is most at risk of cancer?

Fair, red headed, and freckled.

What factors contribute to the prognosis of skin cancer?

1. Grade (based on histology)
2. Stage
3. Site
4. Type and subtype of tumour
5. Thickness and depth (Breslow score, see below)
6. Solitary vs. multiple
7. Associated features (itching, bleeding, recent ↑size).

MALIGNANT MELANOMA

What is malignant melanoma?

Cancer of melanocytes.

So they can be derived from moles?

Yes.

What age group is affected?

20–40 years old.

What is the sex prevalence?

Females > Males.

How may a patient present?

1. Irregular pigmented lesion
2. Rapid increase in size of a pre-existing lesion
3. Itchy lesion
4. Ulceration
5. Satellite nodules.

What are satellite nodules?	Smaller nodules occurring around the primary melanoma, indicating spread.
How can the risk factors of a mole be remembered?	*mnemonic:* **ABCDE** **A**symmetry **B**order irregularity **C**olour variegation (varying colours) **D**iameter (>6 mm is characteristic) **E**volving (ongoing changes)
What types of MM are there?	*mnemonic:* **M**elanoma **A**lways **S**preads to **N**odes (in order of worsening prognosis): *Lentiginous **Maligna:*** macular dark brown/blue lesions, occurs on **face**, neck and arms (skin-exposed areas) ***A**cral Lentiginous:* occur in palms, soles and nail beds; common in dark-skinned races ***S**uperficial spreading:* **most common (70%)**; flat, brown/variegate, occurs on legs, women > men ***N**odular:* dark black/brown dome-shaped nodule which may ulcerate; occurs on trunk and legs; may be amelanotic.
What is lentigo maligna also known as?	A **Hutchinson's freckle** if non-invasive.
How is MM staged?	2 main staging systems exist: **Breslow thickness:** tumour thickness is measured from the most superficial to the deepest point of invasion (mm). **Clarke's levels:** takes into account the anatomical level of skin invaded by the tumour.
What are Clarke's levels?	*mnemonic:* **F**reckles **R**equire **J**udicious **P**athological **E**valuation; from deep to superficial, deep levels having a poorer prognosis:

Fat (Level V; worst prognosis: 75% chance recurrence at 5 years)
Reticular dermis (Level IV)
Junction of reticular and papillary dermis (Level III)
Papillary dermis (Level II)
Epidermis (Level I; best prognosis: approaches 100% chance cure with excision).

What is Breslow's classification?

<0.76 mm has best prognosis (90% chance of cure with excision)
>4 mm has worst prognosis (80% chance recurrence at 5 years).

Which indicator is more reliable?

Breslow's thickness.

Does melanoma metastasise?

Yes!

Where to?

Lymphatic: local and regional lymph nodes; distant skin sites
Haematogenous: small bowel, lung, liver, bone, heart, brain, adrenals.

What are the investigations?

Blood investigations: LFTs (may be ↑ if mets to liver via small bowel)
Imaging:
1. CXR: lung mets
2. CT/MRI for staging if mets suspected only.
Other: sentinel node biopsy can be performed if regional spread suspected only.

What is the treatment?

For *localised disease*, **surgical excision** is performed. Lymph node excision is performed if local or regional spread is present.

What about metastases?

Depends on where to:
Small bowel: resection of affected segment

Lung: resection *if solitary*
Adrenal: resection *if solitary*
Brain: radiation.
In the case of multiple mets, treatment is **palliative**.

Any other modes of treatment?

Adjuvant therapy – Interferon-α2b is under trial. Radio- and chemotherapy have generally poor results.

What are the differential diagnoses of MM?

Atypical mole (syn. **dysplastic naevus**)
Basal cell carcinoma
Squamous cell carcinoma
Dermatofibroma
Keloid or hypertrophic scar
Keratoacanthoma
Seborrhoeic keratosis
Lentigo
Metastatic carcinoma of the skin
Spitz naevus
Vitiligo.

Is the skin the only primary site for melanoma?

No. The eye and anus can also be affected.

SQUAMOUS CELL CARCINOMA

What is SCC?

A malignant tumour of the keratinocytes.

What age groups are affected?

Middle-aged and elderly.

What areas are commonly affected?

Sun exposed areas.

What is the sex prevalence?

F:M = 2:1.

How can a patient present?

1. Newly enlarging lesion which may be bleeding or tender
2. Bleeding
3. Pain
4. Tenderness
5. Personal history of SCC

	6. Family history of SCC
	7. Long history of sun exposure.
What features indicate an aggressive clinical course?	1. Location
	2. Size
	3. Depth of invasion
	4. Level of differentiation
	5. Immunosuppression
	6. Recurrent SCC.
What treatment options are available?	1. Radiotherapy
	2. Cryosurgery
	3. Curettage and electrodesiccation
	4. Excision with conventional margins (4 mm margins)
	5. Mohs micrographic surgery.
What is Mohs micrographic surgery?	Tumour is excised at 45° to the skin piecemeal, and immediately examined under the microscope by a histopathologist. Excision continues until specimens are cleared of tumour by the histopathologist.
What are the differential diagnoses of SCC?	**Basal cell carcinoma**
	Keratoacanthoma
	Actinic keratosis
	Atypical fibroxanthoma
	Pyoderma gangrenosum
	Warts (genital and non-genital).
What is a Marjolin ulcer?	Squamous carcinoma which develops most commonly in **chronic, long-standing venous ulcers**, but can also occur in old scars and osteomyelitic sinuses.

BASAL CELL CARCINOMA

What is BCC?	Malignancy of pluripotent cells in the basal layer of the skin.
What age group(s) is affected?	Adulthood and elderly population.

What areas are commonly affected?	Chronically sun exposed areas (face, scalp, ears, upper trunk).
What is the sex prevalence?	M:F = 3:2
How can BCC present in clinic?	1. Non-healing sore 2. Bleeding with mild trauma 3. Chronic history of sun exposure
What types of BCC are there?	1. Nodular 2. Pigmented 3. Cystic 4. Superficial 5. Micronodular 6. Morphoeaform 7. Infiltrating.
What treatment options are available?	1. Radiotherapy 2. Cryosurgery 3. Curettage and electrodesiccation 4. Excision with conventional margins (to clinically normal skin) 5. Mohs surgery
What are the differential diagnoses of BCC?	**Squamous cell carcinoma** Bowen's disease Actinic keratosis Keratoacanthoma Seborrhoeic keratosis Fibrous papule of the face Melanotic naevi Sebaceous hyperplasia Trichoepithelioma

CHAPTER 50: LYMPHOMAS AND SARCOMAS

What is a lymphoma?
A family of cancers originating from the reticuloendothelial (RES) and lymphatic systems.

What are the two major types of lymphomas?
Hodgkin's and non-Hodgkin's lymphoma (NHL).

HODGKIN'S LYMPHOMA

Who gets Hodgkin's lymphoma?
Bimodal age distribution of peaks at 15–34 and over 60.

Which viruses are associated with it?
Epstein–Barr virus (EBV) and HIV.

What is the pathological hallmark of Hodgkin's disease?
Diagnosis is based upon the finding of Reed–Sternberg cells in the lymph nodes on microscopy. These are large bi-nucleated cells, giving the cells an **'owl's eyes appearance'**. The cells are positive for CD15 and CD30.

What are the signs and symptoms of Hodgkin's disease?
Depends on site and size of node enlargement. **Cervical or mediastinal lymphadenopathy:** can result in nerve compression, causing:
1. Horner's syndrome (compression of cervical sympathetic plexus, causing ipsilateral ptosis, miosis, enophthalmos, and anhidrosis)
2. Laryngeal nerve palsy (causing hoarseness)
3. Neuralgic pain.
Bone marrow: causing bony pain or pancytopenia.
Unusual sites of spread include:
Hepatic ducts: jaundice.
Lymphatics: can result in limb oedema 2ry to lymphatic obstruction.

What are systemic symptoms that occur?
1. Weight loss
2. Fever
3. Night sweats.

These symptoms cause lymphoma to mimic other diseases such as TB, infectious disease and other cancers.

What are these symptoms known as?

B symptoms (see Ann Arbor staging below).

What is the fever associated with Hodgkin's known as?

Pel–Ebstein fever: a few days of fever alternating with days/months of normal temperature.

What are the clinical findings?

General: cachexia and anaemia; may be febrile and/or jaundiced; **painless** cervical lymphadenopathy. *Abdomen:* hepatosplenomegaly.

What are the investigations?

Blood investigations:
1. FBC: normocytic anaemia, ↓ lymphocyte count
2. ↑ ESR
3. LFTs: ↑ ALP due to bone marrow or liver involvement.

Imaging:
1. **CXR:** mediastinal widening 2ry to lymph node involvement, with possible lung involvement.
2. **CT scan:** chest and abdomen for staging of the lymphoma.

Other:
1. **Bone marrow aspirate:** r/o bone marrow involvement.
2. **Lymph node excision biopsy:** Reed–Sternberg cells and CD15/CD30 analysis.

What is a staging laparotomy?

A diagnostic, elective laparotomy performed in an attempt to stage the lymphoma. Rarely done now as it has largely been replaced by CT scan.

Briefly outline the Ann Arbor staging system?

Stage I   Single lymph node region involved.

Stage II   Two or more regions above *or* below the diaphragm.

	Stage III	Involvement of nodes above *and* below the diaphragm.
	Stage IV	Extra-lymphatic spread, eg to the liver, bone marrow.
	B	This is added to any stage if patients also experience B symptoms of fever, weight loss and night sweats.

What is the treatment?

Treatment of choice is radiotherapy with cycles of chemotherapy as this can be **curative**. The exact regime is dependent on the stage and sites of involvement.
Stage I: 80% are disease free at 5 years.
Stage IV: 50% are disease free at 5 years.

What do these patients die from?

Both cell and humoral immunity is depressed leading to bacterial, viral, fungal and protozoan infections, and ultimately sepsis and death.

NON-HODGKIN'S LYMPHOMA (NHL)

What are non-Hodgkin's lymphomas (NHL)?

These are lymphomas with a variety of histological subtypes and are more common than Hodgkin's disease.

Which viruses are thought to be causative factors in the development of NHL?

EBV, HTLV-1 (human T-cell lymphoma virus), and HIV.

Outline a classification system?

1. High grade
2. Intermediate grade
3. Low grade.
This classification is based on the rate of cell replication. They can be further divided into B-cell or T-cell, depending on the cell of origin.

Give examples of these lymphomas	*High grade:* **Burkitt's lymphoma:** first described in African children with reduced immunity 2ry to chronic malarial infection; classically presents as **jaw-line swelling** (endemic or African Burkitt's lymphoma). In Western world, may present as abdominal swelling first, but can affect eyes, ovaries, kidney, breast, thyroid and tonsils (extra-nodal involvement more common). Very strong EBV link; characteristic translocation between chromosome 8 & 14 involving the c-*myc* oncogene. *Intermediate grade:* **Diffuse large cell lymphoma** *Low grade:* the following: 1. **Follicular lymphoma:** B-cell lymphoma occurring in older people, has a chromosome 14 & 18 translocation which over-expresses bcl-2) 2. **Lymphoplasmacytoid lymphoma (Waldenstrom's macroglobulinaemia):** results in an ↑ in monoclonal IgM and a hyperviscosity syndrome.
What are the signs and symptoms of NHL?	These are dependent on the type. There can be peripheral nodal involvement with systemic upset, however, extra-nodal involvement (skin, bone, gut, CNS) is a lot more common and widespread than in Hodgkin's disease.
What are the investigations?	**Blood investigations:** similar to those seen in Hodgkin's lymphoma (see above). Other changes will reflect organ involvement (eg renal failure with altered U+Es may be

apparent if there is nodal obstruction of the ureters).

Imaging:
1. **CXR:** may show mediastinal widening.
2. **CT scan:** shows extent of disease.

Other: a histological diagnosis is essential in NHL. There is an absence of Reed–Sternberg cells. Usually the normal lymphoid architecture and capsule has been destroyed. Immunological studies will suggest a NHL subtype.

What are the treatment options?

Low-grade: localised lymphoma can have radiotherapy alone.

High-grade/advanced disease: may benefit from a combination of chemo- and radiotherapy, or intensive chemotherapy.

These regimes offer a 5-year survival rate of 50–90% depending on regime, subtype (stage/spread) and patient profile.

Should the patient not respond or relapse, autologous stem cell transplantation may be considered.

SARCOMAS

What are sarcomas?

These are tumours of connective tissue (mesenchyme) ie bone, muscle, fat and blood vessels.

How common are they?

Sarcomas are uncommon but can occur in both children and adults.

List some sarcomas

1. Malignant fibrous histocytoma: common in the elderly
2. Fibrosarcoma: arises from fibrocytes; **desmoid tumour** is a form of fibrosarcoma that only spreads to nearby structures.

3. Rhabdomyosarcoma: arises from skeletal muscle. The embryological variety occurs in children while the alveolar type is seen in young adults.
4. Leiomyosarcoma: arises from smooth muscle.
5. Kaposi's sarcoma: arises from endothelial cells. Can effect the skin, mouth, lymph nodes, liver, spleen and lungs. Is associated with HIV, and certain Jewish and eastern European communities.
6. Osteosarcoma: arises from osteocytes and is the second commonest bone tumour.

What causes sarcomas?

Generally, cause is unknown. May be associated with syndromes such as:
1. AIDS
2. Gardner's syndrome (see Chapter 30a)
3. Li–Fraumeni syndrome (p53 mutations)
4. von Recklinghausen's disease (neurofibromatosis).

Radiotherapy and chemical toxins such as vinyl chloride can also cause them.

How may a sarcoma present?

Depends on site and size of sarcoma but are generally painless until they reach a certain size.
- Often they are found on limbs
- Sarcomas of the lung may produce cough and breathlessness
- Uterine sarcoma (a leiomyosarcoma) may produce PV bleeding
- Abdominal sarcomas may produce signs of obstruction.

Do sarcomas spread to lymph nodes?	Rarely (<3%)!
What must be obtained to make a diagnosis?	Tissue biopsy for histopathology.
How is it staged?	The stage is determined by: 1. Size of the tumour (>5 cm associated with a poorer prognosis) 2. Histologic grade (well, moderately, or poorly differentiated) 3. Spread to lymph nodes (very poor prognostic sign) or distant sites.
What are the treatment options?	They are as follows: 1. Surgical excision with negative tissue margins of several centimetres in all directions. 2. Conservative surgical excision with preoperative or postoperative radiation therapy. 3. If the tumour is unresectable, high-dose preoperative radiation therapy may be used, followed by surgical resection and postoperative radiation therapy.
What is GIST?	GastroIntestinal Stromal Tumour. Can occur anywhere along the GI tract but are mainly found in the stomach. Is found in older people and is thought to be caused by a defect in cellular **tyrosine kinase**.
How does GIST present?	Depends on site of GIST in the GI tract, but in general: 1. Abdominal pain 2. Vomiting 3. PR blood 4. May present with acute obstruction.

Once a biopsy is taken how can GIST be diagnosed?

Look for altered expression of tyrosine kinase.

What is the treatment of choice for GIST?

Surgery with adjuvant chemotherapy or radiotherapy. Chemotherapy includes tyrosine kinase inhibitors.

INDEX